2024 Ed

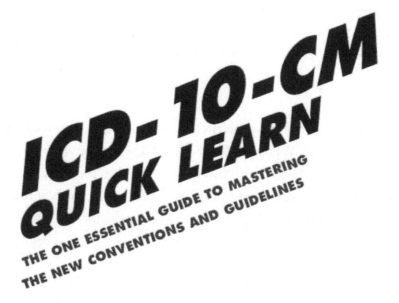

ICD-10-CM
QUICK LEARN
THE ONE ESSENTIAL GUIDE TO MASTERING THE NEW CONVENTIONS AND GUIDELINES

Randall A. Simmons, M.Ed., CRCR

Disclaimer

Nothing in this work should be construed as suggesting that Quick Learn Guides are related to the ICD-10, WHO or NCHS. The ICD-10 is copyrighted by the World Health Organization (WHO), which owns and publishes the classification. ICD-10-CM was developed for use in the United States by The National Center for Health Statistics (NCHS). This Federal agency is responsible for use of the ICD-10 in the United States.

The publisher and the author make no representations or warranties with respect to the accuracy or completeness of the contents of this work. The author warrants that he is not a trained medical professional and nothing in this work should be considered medical advice. Furthermore, nothing in this work should be construed as suggesting that a particular payer will adhere to anything mentioned in this book. Each insurance company and medical payer has its own processing and reimbursement guidelines. Please contact each individual payer to determine its procedures and guidelines in determining reimbursement.

ISBN: 978-0-9970874-0-6

10 9 8 7 6 5 4 3 2 1

The don't-sweat-it style of learning
that cuts to the chase and makes learning fun

ICD-10 requires new learning and this book makes it easy and fun. With over 70,000 codes and thousands of medical and anatomical terms, ICD-10 is a huge challenge. You'll need both a solid understanding of the rules and plenty of practice to master the skill of coding. It's serious business, but there's no rule saying you can't enjoy the process.

Let's Cut to the Chase
Other books spend page after page telling you things you don't need to know. Why waste time learning the history of coding if you don't need it on the job? *ICD-10-CM Quick Learn* focuses on what you need to know.

Forget Memorization!
The format of this book makes it easy to learn without struggle or rote memorization. With its combination of humor, interesting graphics, and lots of interaction, *ICD-10-CM Quick Learn* helps you retain what you learn as effortlessly as possible.

Don't-Sweat-It. Think of It as a Game
By the end of this book you'll know how to use the ICD-10-CM. Plus you'll be shocked to realize that you've learned to recognize hundreds of common medical terms based on their Greek and Latin origins, and be able to figure out long intimidating names of diseases and diagnoses. You'll laugh out loud at some of the crazy sounding codes that the World Health Organization has come up with (you won't believe the codes on page 174). You'll enjoy the scenario-based exercises and doing the detective work to find the appropriate codes. Practice is the easiest way for a motivated student to become proficient quickly and *ICD-10-CM Quick Learn* makes practice fun.

You'll learn more quickly by doing the exercises. In fact, by using this method of learning, you do not need to stress over getting every correct answer the first time. Give it your best shot, but don't sweat it.

Acknowledgements

My sincerest thanks to everyone who contributed to this work. In particular I would like to thank Monica Wurstle for early feedback and Kira Pirre for proofreading assistance.

A special thanks to gifted illustrator Margie Olsen.

And, a very special acknowledgment and a huge thanks to Karen T. Bartlett for her encouragement, support, editing, design and marketing expertise and much more. Without you I would most certainly have suffered from F43.0.

Visit

quicklearnguides.com

for more information, the latest details and to inquire about quantity discounts.

Also Available:

Medical Terminology Quick Learn
The Easiest Guide to
Mastering Basic Medical Terminology
&
Medical Coding Quick Learn
The Easiest Guide to
Mastering Basic Medical Procedure Coding

Contents

About the author

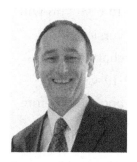

In his three decades of experience in the healthcare reimbursement business, Randall A. Simmons, M.Ed., CRCR, has worked on both the provider side and the payer side.

After earning a Bachelor of Science in psychology, Mr. Simmons earned a Master of Education in instructional technology. He also holds the Certified Revenue Cycle Representative certification from the Healthcare Financial Management Association.

After gaining more than a decade of experience in the insurance industry, Mr. Simmons established his own software company and developed proprietary software to process health insurance claims. He went on to develop computer and internet-based training programs for medical providers, as well as for large and small health insurance companies in North America and abroad.

Mr. Simmons has taught in both the academic environment as a college workforce development instructor and at the corporate level in the medical and insurance fields. He also has developed numerous handbooks, guides and other teaching tools.

Mr. Simmons brings his unique classroom manner to the printed page, making learning easy and fun. And most importantly, his teaching is designed to enable those new to the field, as well as experienced professionals, to become high performers in their chosen careers.

How it works

This **Quick Learn Guide** requires you to practice using the ICD-10-CM. You will need access to an ICD-10-CM code book. You can buy a printed version or download a free electronic version at https://www.cdc.gov. The chapters in this book follow the chapters in the ICD-10. So, Chapter 1 of the ICD-10, Certain Infectious and Parasitic Diseases, is covered in Chapter 1 of this book. But before you start, it's critical to read and do the exercises in Basic Concepts!

After you study the introduction to each chapter in this **Quick Learn Guide**, you'll move directly into practice exercises. The questions are on the front of the page and the answers are on the back often with extra explanations.

Front of page:

4.28
The doctor tells her patient, Jonathan, that he has a diagnosis of type 2 diabetes mellitus with diabetic neuropathic arthropathy. Complete the code for this diagnosis.

E11.*610*

4.29
You see a claim that has both E06.1 and E06.3 used together. Which type of note indicates that this is coded incorrectly?

✓ Excludes1   _____ Excludes2

_____ "Use additional code"   _____ "Code first"

Back of page:

4.28
The complete code for *Type 2 diabetes mellitus with diabetic neuropathic arthropathy* is E11.610.

The codes that begin with E11 are for type 2 diabetes mellitus. Type 1 diabetes mellitus codes begin with E10.

4.29
There is an **Excludes1** note that indicates these two codes should not be used together.

Find E06.1 in your book. Take special note of the **Excludes1** note that mentions E06.3. This means that these two codes should not be used together.

Chapter Quizzes

Each chapter ends with matching exercises or fill in the blank exercises for additional practice. The answers to these exercises are in Appendix A at the back of the book.

NOTE: These quizzes are to give you practice in finding the correct codes and using the rules and conventions of ICD-10-CM. Some exercises may not directly apply to the specialty you are in, but working all of the exercises will greatly enhance your learning of how ICD-10-CM works.

Match the code to the block title the code is in.

_____ 14.21 N21.1	A. Other disease of the urinary system
_____ 14.22 N62	B. Inflammatory diseases of female pelvic organs
_____ 14.23 N45.2	C. Glomerular diseases
_____ 14.24 N13.721	D. Intraoperative and postprocedural complications and disorders of genitourinary system, not elsewhere classified
_____ 14.25 N87.1	E. Acute kidney failure and chronic kidney disease
_____ 14.26 N28.81	F. Diseases of male genital organs
_____ 14.27 N70.13	G. Urolithiasis
_____ 14.28 N35.010	H. Renal tubule-interstitial diseases
_____ 14.29 N04.2	I. Disorders of breast
_____ 14.30 N18.3	J. Other disorders of kidney and ureter
_____ 14.31 N99.510	K. Noninflammatory disorders of female genital tract

x

Quick Quiz

Quick Quizzes will help you remember information covered previously. You'll find the answers in Appendix A. These exercises are meant to reinforce your new knowledge of rules, guidelines and definitions in the ICD-10.

QUICK QUIZ Answers in Appendix A	
____ 2.1 The codes should never be used at the same time	A. Etiology/manifestation
____ 2.2 You must use a different code, but can be used at the same time	B. Excludes1 notes
____ 2.3 Gives examples of content in a category	C. Excludes2 notes
____ 2.4 Tells you that the underlying condition should be coded first	D. Includes notes

There's a code for that??

The ICD-10 includes many unique and sometimes downright hilarious-sounding diagnoses. Throughout the **Quick Learn Guide** we've highlighted a few of these just for fun, and to give your mind a quick break. For example:

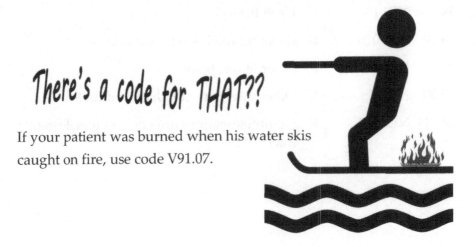

There's a code for THAT??

If your patient was burned when his water skis caught on fire, use code V91.07.

Take Note

Wherever you see the Take Note symbol, you will find important reminders of ICD-10 rules and key information. This information is well worth your time to read and remember.

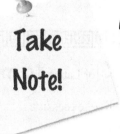

ICD-10 requires you to list the underlying disease (the cause) first, and then list the manifestation.

Hot Tip

A HOT TIP is a professional level insight that will help make you an expert coder.

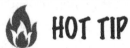 **HOT TIP**

Incorrect use of 7th characters can get your claim processed incorrectly or possibly denied. Become a 7th character expert and you're on your way to being best in the field!

Half-Time and Final Reviews

You'll be amazed at your progress when you work the exercises in the half-time review and the final review. The answers are in Appendix A.

It's all Greek [or Latin] to me!

ICD-10-CM Quick Learn contains more than 200 of the most common Greek and Latin word parts used in medicine. Since diagnoses involve medical terminology, learning some medical terms makes using the ICD-10 quicker and easier. Therefore, as you learn ICD-10 coding with this **Quick Learn Guide**, you will be learning some of the most common medical terms you are likely to see on the job.

When new medical terminology is introduced, whether a prefix, suffix or root word, it is accompanied by a quick reference info box such as the one shown here.

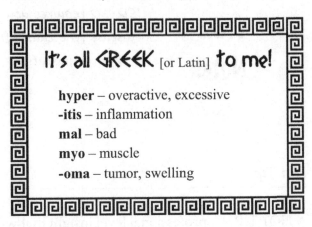

It's all GREEK [or Latin] to me!

hyper – overactive, excessive
-itis – inflammation
mal – bad
myo – muscle
-oma – tumor, swelling

You may have seen medical terms such as cholecystolithiasis, esophagogastroduodenoscopy, or pancreatoduodenostomy. Words like these are unfamiliar to most of us. Do you want to memorize these words and 997 more? Of course you don't. Don't let them scare you. This book **reveals the secret** to identifying and understanding medical terms. You'll be surprised at how many of these words you can absorb quickly and effortlessly as you work through this book. You'll find the Greek and Latin terms covered in this book alphabetized in Appendix B, including the chapter where each one first appears, as in this sample:

-rrhage, abnormal flow or discharge, G, 3	**-stomy**, surgical opening, G, 11
-rrhea, discharge of pus or fluid, G, 8	**sub**, below, L, 6
salping(o), tube, G, 8	**suppuratus**, producing pus, L, 8
scler, hard, G, 7	**syn**, together, G, 17
scoli(o), crookedness, G, 13	**synov**, joint fluid L, 13
sepsis, infection, G, 15	**tachy**, fast, G, 9
sequela, sequel, following, L, 9	**teno**, tendon, G, 13
sial(o), saliva, G, 11	**therm**, heat, G, 16
soma, body, G, 5	**thromb(o)**, clot, G, 3

Conventions used in this book

Chapter Titles

ICD-10-CM chapter titles are capitalized. For example: Diseases of the Digestive System.

Block Numbers

Block numbers are bold. When the official block descriptions follow the number, they will appear in parentheses. For example: **L00-L08** (Infections of the skin and subcutaneous tissue)

Notes

In the **Quick Learn Guide**, the names of notes used in the ICD-10-CM are formatted as follows: **Excludes1, Excludes2, Includes**, **"Code first," "Code also,"** and **"Use additional code."**

Codes and Descriptions

To indicate an official ICD-10-CM code with its full description, the code descriptions are italicized. For example: H92.11 *Otorrhea, right ear.*

Greek and Latin Terms

Greek and Latin terms are shown in ***bold italics*** as in these examples:
Derma- = skin
-itis = inflammation (so dermatitis is inflammation of the skin.)

NOTE: A hyphen after the term indicates that it is being used as a prefix in this case. A hyphen before the term indicates that it is being used as a suffix in this case. Certain word parts can appear as prefixes, suffixes or somewhere in the middle of a medical term.

Information for instructors

While it is a superior self-learning guide for students on their own, *ICD-10-CM Quick Learn* also is an exceptional auxiliary tool for teachers in the classroom environment. Several learning strategies are combined to make this the easiest and most interesting way for students to gain and retain critical knowledge and give them practical experience from the very beginning. The approach is informal and friendly with a variety of scenario based practice exercises that keep the student fully engaged. The exercises are followed by immediate feedback. Scenario-based questions add interest and keep the student's attention. Important information is reviewed several times in varying formats including Quick Quizzes and Chapter Quizzes, eliminating the need for rote memorization and repetitiveness utilized in older style textbooks. With the exception of review exercises, students are never presented more than seven questions without receiving feedback in keeping with the rule of thumb known as Miller's law.

Basic Concepts explains the structure and conventions in the ICD-10-CM code book. Each chapter in *ICD-10-CM Quick Learn* exactly follows the chapters in the ICD-10-CM by chapter number and name. Teachers may choose to use the Half-Time Review and Final Review as exams, or the review questions can form the basis of instructor-generated tests.

This **Quick Learn Guide** can be used in the classroom, assigned as homework, or a combination of the two methods. To help place the terms and information into the student's long-term memory, it is suggested that students concentrate on one chapter at a time. Each chapter reviews and builds upon the important information contained in the prior chapters; a method which has been proven to enhance retention of the material.

The weakness in medical coding study guides currently on the market is that they fill space with extraneous text. *ICD-10-CM Quick Learn* focuses on the "need to know" rather than the "nice to know." This book combines humor, illustrations and a high-level of interaction, combining repetition with novelty in order to maximize learning.

Basic Concepts

ICD-10-CM (also referred to as simply ICD-10, which we will do here) is a list of diagnosis codes for use by hospitals, medical practices and insurance companies. The abbreviation ICD-10-CM stands for International Classification of Diseases - version 10 - Clinical Modification. The codes were adopted in the United States as of October 1, 2015. Throughout this course you'll be working with your ICD-10 code book, in either the printed or electronic version.

If diagnosis coding was easy, you wouldn't need this, or any other, course. You could just look up a code and that would be it. But there are many rules and procedures you must follow. This Guide will teach you the basics in an organized fashion. As you progress through the Guide, the information builds upon what you learned previously. By the time you finish *ICD-10-CM Quick Learn*, you will be well on your way to being an expert coder.

The major sections of the ICD-10 include the following: a tabular listing of the codes divided into 21 chapters, an alphabetical index of diseases and injuries, an alphabetical index of external causes of injuries, the Table of Neoplasms, and the Table of Drugs and Chemicals. Each publisher can put the ICD-10 book in different formats. For example, the sections may be in different order or color coding may be used depending on the publisher. No matter what the publisher's format, the codes used in the ICD-10 system follow a logical and consistent pattern to make coding easier.

If you do not know the code for a disease or condition, you can look it up in the alphabetical index. Then you must verify the code in the tabular listing in the appropriate chapter. It's necessary to always verify the code(s) in the tabular listing, as the index may not provide the full code. In addition, many codes include notes in the tabular listing to help you with the coding. You will learn about these notes as you progress in this guide.

On the next page we will begin our look at the organization of the codes.

THE ABCs OF ICD-10

There are 21 chapters in the ICD-10, categorized by alphanumeric codes A-Z as shown below (Note that there is currently no "U" chapter). All codes in the ICD-10 begin with a letter. The letter is the major classification of diseases. These classifications can be a body system, type of disease, or other classification. The letter and classifications are listed below by chapter name:

A and **B** = Chapter 1: Certain Infectious and Parasitic Diseases

C and **D** = Chapter 2: Neoplasms

D is also in Chapter 3: Diseases of the Blood and Blood-forming Organs

E = Chapter 4: Endocrine, Nutritional and Metabolic Diseases

F = Chapter 5: Mental, Behavioral, and Neurodevelopmental Disorders

G = Chapter 6: Diseases of the Nervous System

H = Chapter 7: Diseases of the Eye and Adnexa

H is also in Chapter 8: Diseases of the Ear and Mastoid Process

I = Chapter 9: Diseases of the Circulatory System

J = Chapter 10: Diseases of the Respiratory System

K = Chapter 11: Diseases of the Digestive System

L = Chapter 12: Diseases of the Skin and Subcutaneous Tissue

M = Chapter 13: Diseases of the Musculoskeletal System

N = Chapter 14: Diseases of the Genitourinary System

O = Chapter 15: Pregnancy, Childbirth and the Puerperium

P = Chapter 16: Certain Conditions Originating in the Perinatal Period

Q = Chapter 17: Congenital Malformations, Deformations and Chromosomal Abnormalities

R = Chapter 18: Symptoms, Signs and Abnormal Clinical and Laboratory Findings, Not Elsewhere Classified

S and **T** = Chapter 19: Injury, Poisoning and Certain Other Consequences of External Causes

V, W, X and **Y** = Chapter 20: External Causes of Morbidity

Z = Chapter 21: Factors Influencing Health Status and Contact with Health Services

ANATOMY OF A CODE

ICD-10 codes are organized into one long tabular list, nicely separated into chapters. Each code begins with a letter of the alphabet, and each chapter focuses on one or two letters. Chapter 1 contains the A and B codes; Chapter 2 covers C and some D codes; Chapter 3 finishes D; Chapter 4 covers the E codes and so on.

The base code (called a category) consists of a letter and two numbers.
The numbers in each chapter start with 00 (except for the F codes, which start with F01). So, for example, the first code in Chapter 1 is A00 and the first code in Chapter 4 is E00. As you scroll down the tabular list, you'll see that the numbers get progressively higher. For example, Chapter 4 codes are numbered from E00 to E89. This part of the ICD-10 is very logical and easy to learn. That is, with the exception of the letter U, which ICD-10 skips altogether. So much for logic!

Most chapters focus on a specific body system.
As a simple example, conditions of the eyes are covered in Chapter 7 and conditions of the ears are covered in Chapter 8. Each chapter is subdivided into sections of categories called **blocks**, which lump related diagnoses together.

For example, the first block in Chapter 10, **J00-J06**, covers acute upper respiratory infections, and the next block, **J09-J18**, covers influenza and pneumonia. This is where it gets a little complicated, because ICD-10 has created subcategories that require you to go deeper and define the condition as much as possible. This means that a code can be as simple as the basic three characters or as detailed as seven characters. Don't worry! The purpose of this book is to make it easy – and even fun - to learn how to choose the most appropriate code.

Simple codes (categories)
A three-character code is appropriate only if that category is not further subdivided with indented codes beneath it. For example, take a quick look at J00, the first code in Chapter 10. It is for acute nasopharyngitis, or the common cold. It is not subdivided, so all you need is code J00.

Indented codes

Now, continue down the codes to J45 *Asthma* (see chart below). This category does have indented codes, so J45 is not complete. You must get more specific. Notice that subcategory J45.2 is further subdivided, so neither J45 nor J45.2 is sufficient. The correct code will have two digits to the right of the decimal point.

J45 *Asthma*
    J45.2 *Mild Intermittent asthma*
        J45.20 *Mild intermittent asthma, uncomplicated*
        J45.21 *Mild intermittent asthma with (acute) exacerbation*
        J45.22 *Mild intermittent asthma with status asthmaticus*

Now, continue down to J45.9. It requires even more detail, for a total of six characters. Don't panic, but on the next page we'll talk about a seventh character!

    J45.9 *Other and unspecified asthma*
        J45.90 *Unspecified asthma*
            J45.901 *Unspecified asthma with (acute) exacerbation*
            J45.902 *Unspecified asthma with status asthmaticus*
            J45.909 *Unspecified asthma, uncomplicated*

Review

*ICD-10 is one continuous tabular list, divided into chapters
*Most chapters focus on a specific body system
*Most chapters cover one letter of the alphabet. Some include two letters.
*Chapters are divided into groups called blocks.
*Each block is divided into categories consisting of a letter of the alphabet followed by two numbers. This is the base code.
*Most base codes (categories) have subcategories indented beneath them.
*If there are subcategories, the base code is never a complete code.
*The fewest number of characters in a code is three. The most characters in a code is seven.

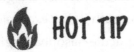

HOT TIP

To save time flipping back to check the letter codes, copy and print
The ABCs of ICD-10 on page 2 and keep it for easy reference.

Placeholders

The letter X is sometimes used as a placeholder character. This is done to allow for future expansion of codes and descriptions. An example of a category with a placeholder character is T39.1X. Find this code in your book. You can see that the codes beneath this category also have the X.

7th character requirements

Some categories require the use of a 7th character, and there will be a note in each category to help you select the valid 7th character. For example, look at code S02, Chapter 19, in your ICD-10. There is a note indicating that a 7th character is required for all the S02 codes, and then the following characters are listed and defined: A, B, D, G, K, and S.

Now look at code S02.101 *Fracture of base of skull, right side.* If the current visit is the initial encounter for a closed fracture, you should add the 7th character A to the end of the code to make it:

S02.101A *Fracture of base of skull, right side, initial encounter for closed fracture*

If this visit is the initial encounter for an open fracture, you will add the 7th character B to the end of the code to give you:

S02.101B *Fracture of base of skull, right side, initial encounter for open fracture*

Likewise, if the current visit is a subsequent encounter for a fracture with routine healing, you would code it:

S02.101D *Fracture of base of skull, right side, subsequent encounter for fracture with routine healing*

Now, look at S02.2 *Fracture of nasal bones.* The 7th character note above it (just under S02) tells you that this code requires a 7th character. Since the code does not already have six characters, you will need to add one or more X's so that you can add the 7th character. This gives us the codes:

S02.2XXA for a *Fracture of nasal bones, initial encounter for a closed fracture,* and
S02.2XXB for a *Fracture of nasal bones, initial encounter for an open fracture*

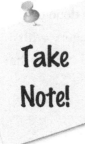

Take Note!

You may need to use more than one X to fulfill the requirement of seven characters. Correct use of placeholders and 7th characters will not only make you a better coder, it can reduce delays in reimbursement.

"Other" and "unspecified"

Codes with "other" in the description are for use when no specific code includes all the detail that is in the doctor's notes. They may be identified as NEC (not elsewhere classifiable). Generally, but not always, "other" codes will have 8 as the last character. For example, look at category K20 *Esophagitis*. Listed beneath it is only one specified code K20.0 *Eosinophilic esophagitis*. Beneath it is K20.8 *Other esophagitis*. This code includes other types of esophagitis besides eosinophilic. Listed below K20.8 is an example, abscess of esophagus.

Codes with "unspecified" in the description are for use when the information in the doctor's notes is not sufficient enough to assign a more specific code. They may be identified as NOS (not otherwise specified). Generally, but not always, "unspecified" codes will have 9 as the last character. For example, K20.9 *Esophagitis, unspecified*. This code is for use when the type of esophagitis is not specified in the doctor's notes.

Multiple codes

You will use as many diagnosis codes as you need to describe the condition(s) or illness(es). Doctors often diagnose more than one condition that needs coding, or you will need to code both the condition and the cause. Many times ICD-10 specifically instructs you to use more than one code.

So, those are some of the basics. Now, let's play around with some chapter exercises. After the overview in each chapter you'll find practice exercises related to that chapter. Look at it as a puzzle and enjoy!

Based on what you've learned so far, give these exercises a try. The answers and explanations are on the next page.

1.

Which of the following statements is true?

_____ Codes consist of only three characters
_____ Codes consist of only seven characters
_____ Codes consist of between three and seven characters

2.

A patient presents with acute mastoiditis. Is H70 an appropriate code for this condition? Hint: look for codes indented beneath H70.

_____ Yes   _____ No

3.

Charley Runinose has a cold. Is J00 the appropriate code for this diagnosis? Look this code up in the J chapter (10) of your ICD-10 book.

_____ Yes   _____ No

4.

Find L03 *Cellulitis and acute lymphangitis* in Chapter 12 of your ICD-10 code book. How are the subcategories broken down?

_____ By time of onset of symptoms   _____ By body part
_____ By mild versus serious   _____ By acute or chronic

Take Note!

This book is designed with the questions on the front of the page and the answers on the back. This is an open book course, but before you flip to the answer, look up the condition in the ICD-10 alphabetical index and it will send you to the appropriate ICD-10 chapter to discover the answer.

1.

Codes consist of between three and seven characters is a true statement.

ICD-10 coding is designed to be used to the highest level of detail; that is, the highest number of characters available. The codes consist of between three and seven characters. Sometimes the basic 3-character code is all that's needed. More often, though, you will find that ICD-10 requires more detail. A 3-character code should be used only if that code is not further subdivided (indented).

2.

No, H70 is not an appropriate code for inflammation of the air cells of the mastoid process. Here's why:

H70 *Mastoiditis and related conditions* is a category and is subdivided. There are codes indented beneath it, such as H70.001 and H70.002. The code with the highest level of detail should be used.

3.

Yes, J00 is the appropriate code for Charley's cold.

J00 is the category for *Acute nasopharyngitis (common cold)*. Notice, however, that the category is not subdivided. This is the only code in the category. Therefore, this is the code to use.

4.

The subcategories for L03 are broken down by body part.

The first level of indentation is for finger and toe, other parts, face and neck, trunk, and other sites. The second level of indentation is also by body part. Look at L03.01 *Cellulitis of finger*. Even the lowest level of this code is by body part. L03.011 is for right finger, L03.012 is for left finger and L03.019 is for unspecified finger. (Unspecified finger??? We didn't write the codes; we just help you learn to use them. "Unspecified" is used only when necessary due to lack of information.)

5.

In the alphabetical index in your ICD-10 code book, find the following condition: goiter due to an enzyme defect in the synthesis of thyroid hormone.
What is the correct code?

_____

6.

Using the alphabetical index in your code book, find thrombophlebitis of the right femoral vein. What is the correct code?

_____

7.

Find acute appendicitis with localized peritonitis in the alphabetical index in your code book. What is the correct code?

_____

8.

Using the alphabetical index in your code book, find unilateral post-traumatic osteoarthritis of the left knee. What is the correct code? Hint: the alphabetical index lists conditions rather than body parts, so start by looking up osteoarthritis.

_____

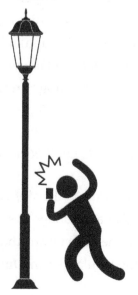

There's a code for THAT??

Code W22.02 is for _Walked into lamppost_.
The patient must have been texting.

5.

<u>E07.1</u> is the code for *dyshormogenetic goiter* (goiter due to an enzyme defect in the synthesis of thyroid hormone).

First, go to the alphabetical index and look up the condition: goiter. There are many entries under goiter. Find the entry for: due to enzyme defect in synthesis of thyroid hormone. Now, look up E07.1 in the tabular list. The description is dyshormogenetic goiter. Notice the **Excludes1** note beneath this code. We will talk more about notes later in this chapter. For now, it is enough to start getting into the habit of looking for notes like this.

6.

<u>I80.11</u> is the code for *Thrombophlebitis of the right femoral vein*.

First, look up the condition thrombophlebitis in the alphabetical index. You will see many entries under thrombophlebitis. Find the entry for femoral vein. The code next to it is I80.1-. The dash means that there are other codes beneath this one. Look up the code in the appropriate chapter in the tabular list. The codes beneath it further clarify which vein. Find the code for right vein: I80.11.

7.

<u>K35.30</u> is the code for *Acute appendicitis with localized peritonitis*.

Look up the condition appendicitis and notice the subdivisions. Look for acute. It, too, has subdivisions. Look for peritonitis and then for localized. The code is K35.30. Next, go to the tabular list, look up the code and check for any notes with this code. As mentioned above, we will cover notes in detail later. For now, just get into the habit of checking before and after each code and see if there are any notes.

8.

<u>M17.32</u> is the code for *Unilateral post-traumatic osteoarthritis of the left knee*.

Find osteoarthritis in the alphabetical index. Look at the subdivisions and you will see post-traumatic. Under post-traumatic you will find knee listed at M17.3-. Remember, the dash means that there are other codes beneath this code. Look up M17.3 in the tabular list and find the code for left knee: M17.32.

Let's get some more practice using the alphabetical index:

9.

Look up acute tracheitis. What is the first letter of the code?

——————

10.

Look up age-related osteoporosis with current pathological fracture of the right shoulder (scapula). What is the first letter of the code?

——————

11.

What is the first letter of the code for sprain of the deltoid ligament of the left ankle?

——————

12.

What is the first letter of the code for acute gastrojejunal ulcer with both hemorrhage and perforation?

——————

13.

You see in the patient's chart a suggested code but you can't read the first letter. However, you can read the description, which is abdominal pregnancy with viable fetus. What is the first letter of the code?

——————

9.

J is the first letter of the code for acute tracheitis.

Look for tracheitis in the alphabetical index, then look for acute. You can see that the code begins with J. The codes that begin with J, as you know from the tabular listing, are in Chapter 10 Diseases of the Respiratory System.

10.

M is the first letter of the code.

Look up the main condition, in this case osteoporosis. Then look for age-related and then "with current pathological fracture." You will then see scapula. The codes that begin with M are for Diseases of the Musculoskeletal System and Connective Tissue.

11.

S is the first letter of the code for sprain of the deltoid ligament of the left ankle.

Look up sprain in the alphabetical index. Under sprain you will see ankle, and under it, deltoid ligament. The code begins with S.

12.

K is the first letter of the code for acute gastrojejunal ulcer with both hemorrhage and perforation.

Look up the primary condition, which is ulcer, in the alphabetical index. Under ulcer, look for gastrojejunal, then acute, then with hemorrhage and perforation. The code begins with K.

13.

O is the first letter of a code for abdominal pregnancy.

In the alphabetical index, look up pregnancy and then find abdominal. The code for abdominal pregnancy with viable fetus is O36.7-. Find it in the tabular list now. You can look down the list and see all pregnancy related codes begin with O.

This time, see if you can answer the following questions using the tabular list within the appropriate chapter:

14.

You see an ICD-10 code on the chart, but you can't read the first letter. The description is major depressive disorder, single episode, severe with psychotic features. What is the first letter of the code? Hint: it's Chapter 5.

_____

15.

You see an ICD-10 code, but you can't read the first letter. The description is congenital cataract. What is the first letter of the code? Hint: cataracts are primarily covered in the eye chapter (7); however, according to the chapter list on page 2 of this **Quick Learn Guide**, congenital conditions are covered in Chapter 17.

_____

16.

You see an ICD-10 code, but you can't read the first letter. The description is staphylococcal scalded skin syndrome. What is the first letter of the code? Hint: the key word is skin.

_____

Take Note!

The ICD-10 is organized into A-Z chapters. The first letter of the code gives you valuable information about the diagnosis. For example, sometimes the first letter of the code tells you which body system is involved. Until you get used to the letters, just flip to the chapter list on page 2 of this **Quick Learn Guide**.

14.

F̲ is the first letter of the code for major depressive disorder, single episode, severe with psychotic features.

Mental, Behavioral, and Neurodevelopmental Disorders begin with F.

The code for *Major depressive disorder, single episode, severe with psychotic features* is F32.3. You can also find it by looking under depression in the alphabetical index, and then going to the chapter indicated to find it in the tabular list.

15.

Q̲ is the first letter of the code for congenital cataract.

ICD-10 codes that begin with Q cover Congenital Malformations, Deformations and Chromosomal Abnormalities. The code for *Congenital cataract* is Q12.0.

16.

L̲ is the first letter of the code for staphylococcal scalded skin syndrome.

Diseases of the Skin and Subcutaneous Tissue, which you will see is Chapter 12, have codes that begin with L.

The code for staphylococcal scalded skin syndrome is L00. You can find it by looking under staphylococcal scalded skin syndrome in the alphabetical index.

Take Note!

ICD-10 consists of a tabular list of 70,000-plus codes divided into chapters. To make it easier for you to find codes there is an alphabetical index. You can look up conditions in the alphabetical index and it will direct you to the code(s) in the tabular list.

Remember, you must always find the code in the tabular list and check for notes.

NOTES: Includes, Excludes, Code Also, and more

We previously talked about "7ᵗʰ **character**" notes. Let's talk about some different types of notes in the ICD-10.

Includes notes

At the beginning of some chapters, after some three-character categories and with some codes beneath the category, you will see an **Includes** note. This note defines the category further, or gives an example of the content of the category.

For example, look at K25. This code is for *Gastric ulcer*. The **Includes** note says that this code is also used for erosion (acute) of stomach, pylorus ulcer (peptic), and stomach ulcer (peptic).

Excludes1 notes

These notes indicate that the code excluded should never be used with this code. The two codes should NOT be used together.

For example, let's look at K25 again. This time, look at the **Excludes1** note. This note tells us that this code can NOT be reported with acute gastritis (K29.0-) and it can NOT be reported with peptic ulcer (K27.-). Notice that the **Excludes1** note even gives us the category for the excluded codes (the dash – indicates that all codes in this category are covered in this note). Remember **Excludes1**=NOT.

Excludes2 notes

This type of note indicates that the condition excluded is not used with this code. It should be given a different code. However, you can use the two together, at the same time. Think **Excludes2** = TOGETHER.

Look at code K22.11. This code is for *Ulcer of esophagus with bleeding*. It has an **Excludes2** note that says "bleeding esophageal varices (I85.01, I85.11)." This means that K22.11 can NOT be used for bleeding of esophageal varices; instead, I85.01 or I85.11 should be used. However, since this is an **Excludes2** note, K22.11 can be coded at the same time as I85.01 or I85.11. Don't worry, this will become easier with practice!

Etiology/manifestation notes

These notes help with the coding of conditions that have both an underlying etiology (the cause) and manifestations (symptoms) due to the underlying etiology. ICD-10 requires you to list the cause first and the manifestation second. The underlying etiology code will have a "**Use additional code**" note. The manifestations codes will have a "**Code first**" note.

Take a look at B20 *HIV* and G05 *Encephalitis, myelitis and encephalomyelitis in diseases classified elsewhere*. After the description of B20 there is a note that says "Use additional code(s) to identify all manifestations of HIV infection." After the description of G05 there is a note that says "Code first underlying disease." Then it lists the diseases you should code first, one of which is *Human immunodeficiency virus [HIV] disease* (B20).

Therefore, the proper order in which to code this combination is:

B20

G05

HIV is the primary disease; it caused the encephalitis; code the HIV first.

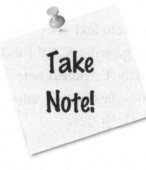

Remember: You must list the underlying etiology (the cause) first, and then list the manifestation.

"Code also" notes

And finally, **"Code also"** notes tell you that another code should be used, but does not require you to put one or the other first. For example, look up code N39.3 *Stress Incontinence (female) (male)*. Notice the **"Code also"** note under it tells you to also use code N32.81 if applicable.

In the following exercises you will practice using some of the notes.

17.

Look at code M80 *Osteoporosis with current pathological fracture* in your code book. Which of these is covered in the **Includes** notes?

_____ Use additional code to identify major osseous defect, if applicable.

_____ Collapsed vertebra NOS

_____ Osteoporosis with current fragility fracture

_____ A 7th character is needed for each code from category M80.

18.

Should H47.611 be coded with S04.041?

_____ Yes   _____ No

19.

Look at code G11. Which condition(s) is/are mentioned in the **Excludes2** note?

_____ Cerebral palsy   _____ Hereditary and idiopathic neuropathy

_____ Metabolic disorders   _____ All of these

20.

Which of these statements is true about **Excludes2** notes?

_____ The two conditions can never be coded at the same time. The codes listed in the **Excludes2** note should never be used with this code.

_____ The patient may have both conditions at the same time and the two codes can be used together.

Take Note!

Notes can cover an entire <u>chapter</u>, or relate specifically to a <u>block</u>, a <u>category</u> or an <u>individual code</u>. You must check all places.

17.

The correct answer is <u>osteoporosis with current fragility fracture</u>.

This code has an **Includes** note, a **"Use additional code"** note, an **Excludes1** note, an **Excludes2** note and a **"7ᵗʰ character"** note.
As you can see, some codes have lots of notes!

18.

<u>No</u>, H47.611 should not be coded with S04.041.

Read the **Excludes1** note associated with H47.6. It says not to code this with S04.04-. Always pay attention to the **Excludes1** notes (and all other notes).

19.

The **Excludes2** note includes <u>all of these</u>.

Cerebral palsy, hereditary and idiopathic neuropathy and metabolic disorders are excluded from the G11 *Hereditary ataxia* category of codes.

20.

The true statement about **Excludes2** notes is: <u>the patient may have both conditions at the same time and the two codes can be used together</u>.

Excludes1 notes mean that the two conditions should never be coded together.
Excludes2 notes mean that the two conditions may be used together, but separate codes should be used.

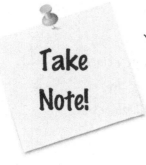

Take Note!

You will save time and avoid unnecessary denials by paying attention to the notes in the ICD-10.

21.

You find it necessary to code M94.351 *Chondrolysis, right hip* and M93.011 *Acute slipped upper femoral epiphysis, stable (nontraumatic), right hip.* Which is the proper sequencing of the codes?

_____ M94.351 and then M93.011   _____ M93.011 and then M94.351

22.

You see a diagnosis code that begins with V. What chapter is this?

_____ Factors Influencing Health Status and Contact with Health Services
_____ External Causes of Morbidity
_____ Symptoms, Signs and Abnormal Clinical and Laboratory Findings

23.

You see a claim, but you can't read the first letter of the ICD-10 code. The description is gastro-esophageal reflux disease with esophagitis. What is the first letter of the code?

_____

24.

You see a claim, but you can't read the first letter of the code. The description is acute recurrent maxillary sinusitis. What is the first letter of the code?

_____

There's a code for THAT??

Accident while playing a musical instrument? Sounds easy, but not so fast! Was it a piano? A drum? A French horn? ICD-10 wants to know. Check out Y93.J-.

21.

<u>M93.011 and then M94.351</u> is the proper sequencing of the codes.

Why? Read the "**Use additional code**" and **"Code first"** notes associated with each category. These are the Etiology/manifestation convention. This convention states that the underlying condition be sequenced first, and then the manifestation. In this case, the acute slipped upper femoral epiphysis is the etiology and chondrolysis is the manifestation.

22.

The <u>External Causes of Morbidity</u> chapter codes begin with V.

In the chapter listing on page 2 you will see that V codes are in Chapter 20. Did you notice that Chapter 20 also has codes that begin with W, X, and Y? Although most chapters have only one letter code, a few chapters have more than one.

23.

<u>K</u> is the first letter of the code for gastro-esophageal reflux disease with esophagitis.

If you don't know the first letter of the code or the chapter number, start by looking up the name of the condition in the alphabetical index. In this case it is reflux. You will see gastroesophageal under reflux. The index gives you the code. Digestive system codes in the ICD-10 begin with K. The complete code for *Gastro-esophageal reflux disease with esophagitis* is K21.0.

24.

J is the first letter of the code for acute recurrent maxillary sinusitis.

Start with the alphabetical index and look for the condition, which is sinusitis. Sinusitis is a disease of the respiratory system. Respiratory system codes in the ICD-10 begin with J. The complete code for *Acute recurrent maxillary sinusitis* is J01.01.

Is it beginning to make sense? Good! Let's review and look closer.

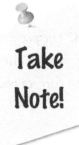

Take Note!

If you don't know which chapter covers the diagnosis you need to code, start with the alphabetical index. Once you get to the chapter you'll see that each level of indentation takes you to a more specific diagnosis.

Let's look at our earlier sample, category J45, again. J tells you this is a disease of the respiratory system, Chapter 10. (Refer back to the chart on page 2). So, any time you see an ICD-10 code that begins with J, you know that it's a disease of the respiratory system. After the letter, there is a two-digit number. In our example the number is 45. In this case, the two-digit number is the disease, which is asthma.

Now look at J45 in your ICD-10 book. You will see that it is further broken down into subcategories by severity of the disease, as follows.

> J45.2 *Mild intermittent*
> J45.3 *Mild persistent*
> J45.4 *Moderate persistent*
> J45.5 *Severe persistent*
> J45.9 *Other and unspecified*

But you're still not finished. Asthma codes have another level of indentation. You'll see that J45.2 is divided into:

> J45.20 *Mild intermittent asthma, uncomplicated*
> J45.21 *Mild intermittent asthma with (acute) exacerbation*
> J45.22 *Mild intermittent asthma with status asthmaticus*

Now look at code J45.90. You will see that it's subdivided even further:

> J45.901 *Unspecified asthma with (acute) exacerbation*
> J45.902 *Unspecified asthma with status asthmaticus*
> J45.909 *Unspecified asthma, uncomplicated*

Always use the most detailed, specific code (the one with the most characters for the condition you are coding) based on the patient's chart.

Remember, not all categories are subdivided. Look at code J42 *Unspecified chronic bronchitis* in your code book. This category does not have any further divisions. In this case, the basic category is all there is. So, J42 would be the correct code to use.

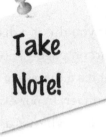

You must select the most specific code available. The indented format makes it easier to read and find codes.

You may only use a three-digit code (category) when there are no indented codes beneath it.

Chapter-Specific Coding Guidelines.

Find the section in your ICD-10 book entitled Chapter-Specific Coding Guidelines. This section explains guidelines that apply to specific chapters. These guidelines can help you find the correct code. For example, if you want to find the guidelines for a certain disease of the eye (which is Chapter 7), you should look in the Chapter-Specific Coding Guidelines section for Chapter 7.

Take a look at the Chapter 7 specific coding guidelines. If the diagnosis involves glaucoma or blindness, these guidelines are very important. However, if the doctor's diagnosis does not involve these, the guidelines won't apply.

Now, look at the Chapter-Specific Coding Guidelines for Chapter 9: Diseases of the Circulatory System. It consists of guidelines for:

a) Hypertension

b) Atherosclerotic coronary artery disease and angina

c) Intraoperative and postprocedural cerebrovascular accident

d) Sequelae of cerebrovascular disease

e) Acute myocardial infarction.

Each of these topics (a-e) contains necessary instructions for correctly coding those diagnoses.

 HOT TIP

One of the most important things you can do is to become familiar with the Chapter-Specific Coding Guidelines. They contain important information that will be critical in selecting the correct code.

There's a code for THAT??

ICD-10 requires you to be specific in coding all those bird bites, strikes, pecks and other injuries!

Under W61, you've got parrots, macaws, psittacines (which are members of the parrot family), chickens, turkeys, geese, ducks and others. Let's hope the patient knows her birds!

HOT TIP

Even if you only code for one or two medical specialties, you will benefit by working through the entire **Quick Learn Guide**. Understand ICD-10 best and be prepared for future career growth.

Are you ready for some practice with the Chapter-Specific Coding Guidelines? Here are a couple of quick exercises.

25.

Look at the Chapter-Specific Coding Guidelines for Chapter 2: Neoplasms. Notice that the first subsection is for "General guidelines." Flip through all the chapters. Do all chapters have a "General guidelines" subsection?

_____ Yes   _____ No

26.

Look at the Chapter-Specific Coding Guidelines for Chapter 15: Pregnancy, Childbirth, and the Puerperium. How many lettered subsections are there?

_____ 18 (a-r)   _____ 3 (a-c)   _____ only 1

QUICK QUIZ *Answers in Appendix A*

_____ 1. External Causes of Morbidity	**A.** Codes begin with C or D
_____ 2. Diseases of the Digestive System	**B.** Codes begin with Y
_____ 3. Neoplasms	**C.** Codes begin with M
_____ 4. Diseases of the Musculoskeletal System	**D.** Codes begin with K

25.

No, not all chapters have a "General guidelines" subsection.

Some chapters have "General guidelines"; others do not.

26.

The number of lettered subsections for Chapter 15 is 18 (a-r).

The chapter on Pregnancy, Childbirth, and the Puerperium has a lot of Chapter-Specific Coding Guidelines. You can see how important it is to familiarize yourself with these notes. You may not memorize all of them, but knowing that they are there and referring to them gives you a huge advantage.

QUICK QUIZ *Answers in Appendix A*

_____ 5. Injuries or Poisoning   **A.** Codes begin with J

_____ 6. Diseases of the Respiratory System   **B.** Codes begin with D

_____ 7. Certain Infectious and Parasitic   **C.** Codes begin with A or B
         Diseases

_____ 8. Diseases of the Blood   **D.** Codes begin with S or T

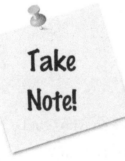

Take Note!

Remember:

EXCLUDES1= codes can NOT be used at the same time

EXCLUDES2= codes can be used TOGETHER

1

Certain Infectious and Parasitic Diseases

Now that we have some basic concepts down, let's begin exploring the individual chapters. All codes in Chapter 1 start with the letter A or B. Each chapter will have its own set of notes at the beginning. Some chapters have many notes while other chapters have only one. In this case there are four notes.

> **Includes** tells you that codes in this chapter are for communicable or
> transmissible diseases.
>
> **"Use additional code"** deals specifically with Z16.
>
> **Excludes1** indicates that certain localized infections should be coded in the
> body system-related chapters.
>
> **Excludes2** lists some conditions that should be coded separately but that
> can be billed at the same time.

Chapter 1 has more than the average Chapter-Specific Coding Guidelines. Such as human immunodeficiency virus (HIV) infections, and infections resistant to antibiotics.

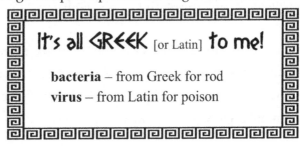

It's all GREEK [or Latin] to me!

bacteria – from Greek for rod
virus – from Latin for poison

Each chapter is divided into sections called blocks. Chapter 1 has 22 blocks. They start with **A00-A09** and end with **B99**. Notice that the codes progress in numerical order. The first several blocks of the A codes are for bacterial conditions, and then viral infections begin with **Block A80-A89**.

The notes at the beginning of each chapter apply to the entire chapter. Some blocks have notes that apply only to that block. In addition, some categories and even some individual codes have notes. Look at **Block A00-A09** (Intestinal infectious diseases), the first block of codes in this chapter, and find A02 *Other salmonella infections*. Read the **Includes** note after this code.

It informs you that the codes indented under A02 include infection or foodborne intoxication due to any Salmonella species other than S. typhi and S. paratyphi.

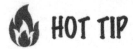

HOT TIP

Even when you're pretty sure of your code, it's smart to take a quick scan of nearby codes. This can help affirm that you are selecting the best code for the particular situation.

Find **Block A20-A28** (Certain zoonotic bacterial diseases) in your ICD-10 and locate code A28 *Other zoonotic bacterial diseases, not elsewhere classified*. You will see codes like this (Other…) throughout the ICD-10 code book. These are "catch-all" codes to be used when no other code is appropriate.

Find code A32 *Listeriosis* in **Block A30-A49** (Other bacterial diseases). Read the notes that apply to the A32 codes. **Includes** tells you that these codes are for listerial foodborne infection. **Excludes1** instructs you not to use P37.2 *Neonatal (disseminated) listeriosis* with the A32 codes.

Take a look at **Block A70-A74** (Other diseases caused by chlamydiae). This block has only three codes and a few indented codes. You will find that some blocks in the ICD-10 contain several pages of codes while other blocks, such as this one, contain only a few (or even just one) code.

Some common viral infections are B00 *Herpesviral [herpes simplex] infections*, B01 *Varicella [chickenpox]*, B05 *Measles*, and B06 *Rubella [German measles]*. All of these codes can be found in the first B block, **B00-B09** (Viral infections characterized by skin and mucous membrane lesions).

Notice that human immunodeficiency virus [HIV] disease has its own block, **B20**. This block contains only one code, but it has four notes. **Includes** informs you of the types of conditions included in this block: acquired immune deficiency syndrome [AIDS], AIDS- related complex [ARC] and HIV infection, symptomatic.

"Code first" tells you to list any O98.7 *Human immunodeficiency virus [HIV] disease complicating pregnancy, childbirth and the puerperium* codes first, if they are applicable. **"Use additional code"** tells you to identify all manifestations of HIV infection. And **Excludes1** lists three codes that cannot be used with B20: Z21 *Asymptomatic human immunodeficiency virus [HIV] infection status*, Z20.6 *Exposure to HIV virus*, and R75 *Inconclusive serologic evidence of HIV*.

Here are some exercises to practice coding Chapter 1.

1.1

A00 *Cholera* is an example of a:

_____ Block   _____ Category   _____ Code

1.2

B87.1 *Wound myiasis* is an example of a:

_____ Block   _____ Category   _____ Code

1.3

At the beginning of Chapter 1 is a list of blocks (sections) within the chapter. Read through the list and find the range of codes for protozoal diseases. What is the correct range of codes?

_____ **B15-B19**   _____ **B50-B64**   _____ **B65-B83**   _____ **B95-B97**

1.4

You see a claim with a diagnosis code of A22.0 *Cutaneous anthrax*. In which block is this included?

_____ Intestinal infectious disease   _____ Tuberculosis

_____ Certain zoonotic bacterial diseases   _____ Other spirochetal diseases

1.1

The first <u>category</u> in this chapter is A00 *Cholera*.

Notice the indented codes beneath cholera. When there are indented codes, the top code is the category and should not be used. Follow the indented codes until you get to the codes with the highest number of characters. You should always use the codes with the most characters. The first code that you should use in this chapter is A00.0.

Take Note!

1.2

B87.1 is an example of a <u>code</u>.

The category above B87.1 is B87 *Myiasis*. The block above B87 is **B85-B89** (Pediculosis, acariasis and other infestations).

In Chapter 1 some codes begin with A and some begin with B. In most chapters of the ICD-10, all the codes begin with the same letter, but there are a few chapters in which codes start with more than one letter as is the case with Chapter 1.

1.3

The range of codes for the protozoal diseases block is <u>**B50-B64**</u>.

Using the list of blocks at the beginning of each chapter is a quick way to find the code you need. Randomly select a few chapters and look at the lists. Did all of the chapters you selected have a list of blocks at the beginning of the chapter? Did you notice that some blocks have **Includes, Excludes** or other notes?

1.4

A22.0 *Cutaneous anthrax* is included in the <u>Certain zoonotic bacterial diseases</u> block.

A22.0 falls between A20 and A28, which make up the block for Certain zoonotic bacterial diseases.

1.5

You see a medical record with a diagnosis of B05.2 *Measles complicated by pneumonia*. In which block is this located?

_____ Arthropod-borne viral fevers   _____ Viral infections characterized by
       & viral hemorrhagic fevers   skin & mucous membrane lesions
_____ Other viral diseases   _____ Mycoses

1.6

The patient's claim has a diagnosis of C02.8. Is this diagnosis under Certain Infectious and Parasitic Diseases?

_____ Yes   _____ No

1.7

Should A51.0 *Primary genital syphilis* be used at the same time as B20, the code for HIV disease? Hint: Don't forget to check the notes at the beginning of each block.

_____ Yes   _____ No

1.8

Based on the **Excludes2** note in the block titled "Other spirochetal diseases," which of the following is true?

_____ It is ok to code A50.01 and A69.1 at the same time
_____ It is NOT ok to code A50.01 and A69.1 at the same time
_____ It is ok to code A50.01 and A69.1 at the same time, but only if certain
       conditions are met

1.9

Find the code A77.40. Under which block is it listed?

_____ Other diseases caused by chlamydiae   _____ Rickettsioses
_____ Viral and prion infections of the central   _____ Other spirochetal
       nervous system   diseases

1.5

B05.2 *Measles complicated by pneumonia* is in the block <u>Viral infections characterized by skin and mucous membrane lesions</u>.

B05.2 falls between B00 and B09, which make up the block for Viral infections characterized by skin and mucous membrane lesions.

1.6

<u>No</u>, C02.8 is not in the Certain Infectious and Parasitic Diseases chapter.

Codes for Certain Infectious and Parasitic Diseases begin with A or B. Codes that begin with C are covered in the next chapter, Neoplasms.

1.7

<u>No</u>, a code for primary genital syphilis should not be used at the same time as a code for HIV disease.

Go to the code for primary genital syphilis: A51.0. It falls under the **Block A50-A64** (Infections with a predominantly sexual mode of transmission). This block has an **Excludes2** note that says the condition excluded (B20) should be given a different code than this one (A51.0) but it is ok to code them at the same time.

1.8

<u>It is ok to code A50.01 and A69.1 at the same time</u> is the correct answer.

How do you know? The **Excludes2** note with the block tells you that the condition excluded (A50.01) should be given a different code than the one listed here (A69.1), but it is ok to use the other code at the same time as this one.

1.9

A77.40 is listed in the block <u>Rickettsioses</u>.

The block Rickettsioses includes codes A75-A79. A77.40 *Ehrlichiosis, unspecified* is indented under A77 *Spotted Fever [tick-borne rickettsioses]*.

1.10

Based on what you've learned about **Excludes1** notes, do you think it is acceptable to bill A49.01 and A74.9 on the same claim?

_____ Yes, billing A49.01 and A74.9 on the same claim is correct

_____ No, code A49.01 should not be billed at the same time as A74.9

1.11

Which of the following codes would NOT be found in Chapter 1?

_____ A18.82   _____ B37.41   _____ B95.2   _____ C04.1

1.12

You see a claim with the diagnosis of Echinococcus granulosus infection, thyroid gland. Enter the digits after the decimal point.

B67._____

1.13

You see a claim with the diagnosis of meningitis due to Lyme disease. Enter the digits after the decimal point.

A69._____

1.14

Look at the note under the **Block B95-B97** (Bacterial and viral infectious agents). Do you think it is appropriate to bill one of these codes by itself?

_____ Yes   _____ No

Take Note!

Notes help you find the correct code and avoid mistakes. Save yourself a re-do by reading the notes!

1.10

No, code A49.01 should not be billed at the same time as A74.9.

Why not? **Excludes1** notes tell you that the two codes should NOT be billed at the same time. The **Excludes1** note under A49 lists chlamydial infection NOS (A74.9). Therefore, A74.9 should not be billed with A49.01.

1.11

C04.1 is not found under Certain Infectious and Parasitic Diseases.

All codes in the chapter for Certain Infectious and Parasitic Diseases begin with either A or B. Codes that begin with C are in Chapter 2, Neoplasms.

1.12

The correct digits are 31.

B67 covers Echinococcosis. It has indents to further specify the type of echinococcosis and the location. So, the complete code is B67.31 *Echinococcus granulosus infection, thyroid gland.*

1.13

The correct digits are 21.

A69 is for Other spirochetal infections. A69.2 is for Lyme disease, and to further define it A69.21 is for *Meningitis due to Lyme disease.*

1.14

No.

Why not? The note at the beginning of the block says these codes are to be used as supplementary or additional codes for diseases classified elsewhere. This means you must use a primary code first.

Chapter Quiz (Answers in Appendix A)

Match the code to the block title the code is in.

_____ 1.1	A40.3	A.	Intestinal infectious diseases
_____ 1.2	A71.0	B.	Tuberculosis
_____ 1.3	B05.9	C.	Certain zoonotic bacterial diseases
_____ 1.4	A82.1	D.	Other bacterial diseases
_____ 1.5	B30.1	E.	Infections with a predominantly sexual mode of transmission
_____ 1.6	B15.9	F.	Other spirochetal diseases
_____ 1.7	A95.0	G.	Other diseases caused by chlamydiae
_____ 1.8	A08.19	H.	Rickettsioses
_____ 1.9	B86	I.	Viral and prion infections of the central nervous system
_____ 1.10	A69.20	J.	Arthropod-borne viral fevers and viral hemorrhagic fevers
_____ 1.11	B76.0	K.	Viral infections characterized by skin and mucous membrane lesions
_____ 1.12	A75.1	L.	Viral hepatitis
_____ 1.13	B20	M.	Human immunodeficiency virus (HIV) disease
_____ 1.14	A17.0	N.	Other viral diseases
_____ 1.15	B96.21	O.	Mycoses
_____ 1.16	A51.0	P.	Protozoal diseases
_____ 1.17	B52.9	Q.	Helminthiases
_____ 1.18	B90.0	R.	Pediculosis, acariasis and other infestations
_____ 1.19	B37.3	S.	Sequelae of infectious and parasitic diseases
_____ 1.20	A27.0	T.	Bacterial and viral infectious agents

Match the chapter to the first letter of the code. NOTE: use H twice!

_____ 1.21	Injuries or Poisoning	A.	Codes begin with A or B
_____ 1.22	Skin and Subcutaneous Tissue	C.	Codes begin with C or D
_____ 1.23	Respiratory System	D.	Codes begin with D
_____ 1.24	Factors Influencing Health Status	E.	Codes begin with E
_____ 1.25	Circulatory System	F.	Codes begin with F
_____ 1.26	Certain Infectious Diseases	G.	Codes begin with G
_____ 1.27	The Perinatal Period	H.	Codes begin with H
_____ 1.28	Mental and Behavioral	H.	Codes begin with H
_____ 1.29	Disease of the Blood	I.	Codes begin with I
_____ 1.30	Digestive System	J.	Codes begin with J
_____ 1.31	Musculoskeletal System	K.	Codes begin with K
_____ 1.32	Endocrine Diseases	L.	Codes begin with L
_____ 1.33	Symptoms and Signs	M.	Codes begin with M
_____ 1.34	Genitourinary System	N.	Codes begin with N
_____ 1.35	Eye and Adnexa	O.	Codes begin with O
_____ 1.36	Nervous System	P.	Codes begin with P
_____ 1.37	Neoplasms	Q.	Codes begin with Q
_____ 1.38	Congenital Malformations	R.	Codes begin with R
_____ 1.39	Ear and Mastoid Process	S.	Codes begin with S or T
_____ 1.40	Pregnancy	Z.	Codes begin with Z

2

Neoplasms

Chapter 2 in the ICD-10 code book covers neoplasms. A neoplasm is an abnormal formation of tissue, also called a tumor. Neoplasms grow at the expense of normal tissue and they serve no purpose. This chapter is especially important because neoplasms can occur in many places throughout the body, so you may use these codes in many specialties.

So, let's take a look at this important chapter. As you will find throughout the ICD-10 book, the blocks are listed at the beginning of the chapter. The first block is **C00-C14** (Malignant neoplasms of lip, oral cavity and pharynx). The last block is **D49** (Neoplasms of unspecified behavior).

You've learned from the chart on page 2 that in most chapters the codes begin with the same letter. But as with Chapter 1, this is not always the case. Did you notice that some codes in Chapter 2 begin with C and others begin with D?

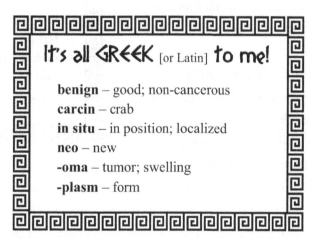

It's all GREEK [or Latin] to me!

benign – good; non-cancerous
carcin – crab
in situ – in position; localized
neo – new
-oma – tumor; swelling
-plasm – form

All of the codes that begin with C are for malignant neoplasms. Malignant means the neoplasm is cancerous. Look at the list of blocks for malignant neoplasms. Notice that they are categorized by body part. The first block is for lip, oral cavity and pharynx, followed by digestive organs, and then respiratory and intrathoracic organs, and so on.

Look at the first block that begins with D: **Block D00-D09**. These codes are for in situ neoplasms. In situ means "in position." When a neoplasm or tumor is localized, or not invading the surrounding tissue, it is said to be "in situ."

Blocks D10-D36 and **D3A** are for benign neoplasms and benign neuroendocrine tumors. Benign means non-cancerous. Benign tumors and neoplasms do not invade neighboring tissues and they are not life threatening.

Let's look at some other terms you will see in Chapter 2. Carcinoma is a type of cancer that develops from epithelial cells, which cover the surface of a body or organ. Find code D00 in your ICD-10 code book. The description is *Carcinoma in situ of oral cavity, esophagus and stomach*. Browse through this block and notice that the codes are conveniently divided by body part.

Mesothelioma (code C45) is a type of cancer that develops in the protective lining of many organs, melanoma (C43) is a type of skin cancer, and lymphoma (C81-C88) is a type of tumor made from lymphocytes. Notice anything similar in all these words? They all end in -*oma*. A medical word that ends in -*oma* refers to a disease in which there is abnormal growth of cells.

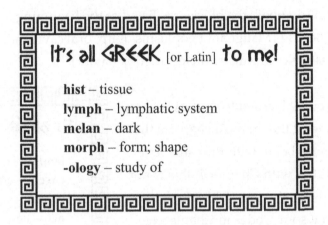

It's all GREEK [or Latin] to me!

hist – tissue
lymph – lymphatic system
melan – dark
morph – form; shape
-ology – study of

In this chapter we've introduced the fun boxes defining basic root words, called It's all Greek [or Latin] to me! Let's look at some of these words in Chapter 2. A medical word that ends in -*ology* means "the study of." Morphology is the study of the form or shape of an organism or even a part of an organism such as the shape of a neoplasm or tumor. Histology is the study of tissues or cells. You will see some of these terms in this chapter.

Are you ready to practice coding in this chapter? Use the pages you just read and check the Greek and Latin terms you just read to answer the following questions.

2.1

A neoplasm could be defined as:

_____ A new tumor or growth

_____ An organ in the digestive system

_____ A type of bacterial infection

2.2

Certain types of neoplasms are malignant (cancerous). Codes for malignant neoplasms start with what letter(s)?

_____ A & B   _____ C   _____ C & D   _____ D

2.3

The codes for benign (non-cancerous) neoplasms start with what letter(s)?

_____ A & B   _____ C   _____ C & D   _____ D

2.4

Polly Sue's doctor has diagnosed her with a type of cancer that develops from epithelial cells. It is code C22.0 in your ICD-10 book. Find code C22.0 and name the type of cancer.

_____ Melanoma   _____ Carcinoma

_____ Mesothelioma   _____ Lymphoma

 HOT TIP

Need to look up the description for a code but don't have a book handy? Just enter the code into your search engine. For example: ICD-10 K40.21.

2.1

A neoplasm is <u>a new tumor or growth</u>.

Neoplasms are abnormal formations of tissue. There are many types of neoplasms.

2.2

The correct answer is <u>C & D</u>.

All C codes are for malignant neoplasms and D codes contain both malignant and benign diagnoses.

2.3

The correct answer is <u>D</u>.

A benign neoplasm is non-cancerous. You cannot use a C code with a benign tumor. The dictionary defines benign as meaning gentle or kind.

2.4

C22.0 is for <u>carcinoma</u>.

Check your Greek and Latin box for the word carcinoma. It comes from Greek *carcin-* meaning crab (or in medical terms a crab-like growth) and refers to cancer and *-oma* means tumor or swelling. By placing *carcin-* in front of *-oma* it means the tumor is cancerous.

QUICK QUIZ *Answers in Appendix A*

_____ 2.1 The codes should never be used at the same time

_____ 2.2 You must use a different code, but can be used at the same time

_____ 2.3 Gives examples of content in a category

_____ 2.4 Tells you that the underlying condition should be coded first

A. Etiology/manifestation

B. **Excludes1** notes

C. **Excludes2** notes

D. **Includes** notes

2.5

Roger has a rare form of cancer called mesothelioma. He worked in a factory with asbestos for 30 years. Go to the category of C45 codes and check the correct code for mesothelioma of the pericardium.

_____ C45.0   _____ C45.1

_____ C45.2   _____ C45.7

2.6

Nikoli loved going to the beach as a child. He would spend all day surfing and lying on the beach. He recently noticed a darkly pigmented mole on his nose. His doctor called it a melanoma. What code will you use?

_____ C43.3   _____ C43.30

_____ C43.31   _____ C43.39

2.7

Lucy's doctor told her she has a follicular lymphoma of the spleen, grade II. What code will you use for this disease?

_____ C82.07   _____ C82.09

_____ C82.17   _____ C82.27

2.8

Code C44.01 identifies the most common type of skin cancer. What is it?

_____ Basal cell   _____ Squamous cell   _____ Hodgkin lymphoma
carcinoma   carcinoma

2.9

C44.02 is a cancer of the main part of the epidermis of the skin. What is it?

_____ Basal cell   _____ Squamous cell   _____ Hodgkin lymphoma
carcinoma   carcinoma

2.5

C45.2 is the code for mesothelioma of the pericardium.

Start with C45 *Mesothelioma*. Now look at the indented codes for pericardium.

2.6

C43.31 is the code for malignant melanoma of the nose.

Start with C43 *Malignant melanoma of skin*. Look at the indented codes for face (C43.3) and then nose. ***Melan-*** comes from the Greek work for dark. As you know, ***-oma*** indicates tumor. A primary cause of melanoma is excessive exposure to ultraviolet light from the sun.

2.7

C82.17 is follicular lymphoma grade II, spleen.

To find the complete code start with follicular lymphoma, which is C82. Beneath that look for grade II, which is C82.1 and then notice that it is further divided by the affected body part

Lymphoma is a type of cancer that occurs in the lymphatic system. When lymphocytes (white blood cells) multiply uncontrollably they produce cancerous cells.

2.8

Basal cell carcinoma is the most common type of skin cancer. It can cause much damage and destruction to surrounding tissues.

2.9

Squamous cell carcinoma affects the main part of the epidermis of the skin.

The squamous cell is the main part of the epidermis of the skin, therefore, squamous cell carcinoma is a type of skin cancer. However, squamous cells occur elsewhere in the body and squamous cell cancer can be found in the lips, lungs and other areas.

2.10

Dr. Able is studying a patient's cells and tissues using an electron microscope. Based on the Greek and Latin root words you've learned so far, what is this called? Hint: see the box on page 38.

_____ Morphology _____ Histology

2.11

For another patient Dr. Able is studying the shape and form of a neoplasm. What is this called?

_____ Morphology _____ Histology

2.12

Block D00-D09 covers in situ neoplasms. What does in situ mean? Hint: see the box on page 37.

_____ Invading the surrounding tissue
_____ Localized in one area and not invading surrounding tissue

2.13

Does this chapter include all codes for both benign and malignant neoplasms? Hint: Check the Chapter-Specific Coding Guidelines for the Neoplasms chapter.

_____ Yes, all benign and malignant neoplasms are included in this chapter
_____ No, not all are included in this chapter

There's a code for THAT??

Just in case there's such a thing as vampires, code S11.85 has you covered! It specifies "open bite of other specified part of neck."

2.10

Histology is the study of tissue or cells.

Histo- comes from the Greek word for tissue and *-ology* comes from the Greek word for science, or the study of something. Scientists can use a light microscope to view tissue or a much more powerful electron microscope to peer into the tiniest parts of a cell.

2.11

Morphology is the study of the form or shape of an organism or a part of an organism such as a neoplasm or tumor.

Morph- comes from the Greek word for form and *-ology* is Greek for the study of something. Put these two together and you have morphology – the study of form or shape.

2.12

In situ means a neoplasm that is localized and not invading the surrounding tissue.

In situ is a term that means "in position." You can think of 'in situ' as 'u sit down'. The tumor is sitting in one place.

2.13

No, not all of the codes for benign and malignant neoplasms are included in this chapter.

How do you know? Because the first sentence in the Chapter-Specific Coding Guidelines says that this chapter includes codes for most, but not all, benign neoplasms and for all malignant neoplasms. Some benign neoplasms are found in the chapter covering the specific body system affected.

2.14

Sometimes you will use more than one code on a claim. In some cases there is a certain order in which you must list the codes. According to the Chapter-Specific Coding Guidelines for Chapter 2, when a neoplasm is removed and an adjunct chemotherapy or radiation treatment is administered in one episode of care, which should be listed as the principle (or first listed) diagnosis?

_____ The removal of the neoplasm
_____ The chemotherapy or radiation treatment

2.15

Read about sequencing of neoplasm codes in the Chapter-Specific Coding Guidelines, and then answer this question: If a patient has a primary malignancy with metastasis and the treatment is only directed toward the metastatic site, which of the following is the principle, or first listed, diagnosis?

_____ The primary site   _____ The metastatic site

2.16

Chapter 2 is broken down into broad categories, listed at the beginning of the chapter. Look at the list and determine how neoplasms are primarily classified.

_____ By location (ie, digestive organ, skin, etc)
_____ By name of neoplasm

 HOT TIP

The ICD-10 has a quick way to look up neoplasms. It is the only condition that has its own table. Locate the Table of Neoplasms and notice that it is ordered by location in the body and then the type. After you find the neoplasm in the table, then read across the page to the type of neoplasm (e.g., benign) and find the code.

2.14

The removal of the neoplasm is the primary diagnosis.

The Chapter-Specific Coding Guidelines for this chapter – guideline e) 1 – states that when a neoplasm is removed (excised) and adjunct chemotherapy or radiation treatment is also done at the same encounter, the removal of the neoplasm should be the principle or primary diagnosis.

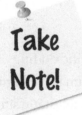

Take Note!

The principle, or primary, diagnosis is the one you should list first.

2.15

The metastatic site is the primary diagnosis.

Find the section of the Chapter-Specific Coding Guidelines titled "Sequencing of neoplasm codes" and then look for "Encounter for treatment of secondary malignancy." It states: When the treatment is on the metastatic site only, the metastatic site should be coded as the principle (first listed) diagnosis.

2.16

Neoplasms are primarily classified by location (i.e., digestive organ, skin, etc).

 HOT TIP

To become an expert coder you must learn some medical terminology. Medical words are often formed by combining two or more Greek or Latin based word parts. The first word part is called the **prefix** and the last part is the **suffix**. For example, *carcin-* is a prefix meaning cancerous and *–oma* is a suffix meaning tumor. When you combine them you get the word carcinoma, cancerous tumor.

2.17

Dr. Able's diagnosis is malignant neoplasm of vestibule of mouth. Complete the code.

C06._____

2.18

Look at the block for malignant neoplasms of digestive organs. What organ is listed first?

_____ Stomach   _____ Small intestine

_____ Colon   _____ Esophagus

2.19

Find the block of codes for malignant neoplasms of thyroid and other endocrine glands. In what order are the glands listed?

_____ Other, adrenal and thyroid

_____ Thyroid, adrenal and other

_____ Adrenal, thyroid and other

2.20

What major code comes after C75?

_____ C76   _____ C7A   _____ C77

There's a code for THAT??

Believe it or not, yes! Check code
Z18.31 *Retained animal quills or spines.*

2.17

The complete code is <u>C06.1</u>.

Did you notice that C06 is for *Malignant neoplasm of other and unspecified parts of the mouth*? Since the doctor specified the vestibule of the mouth, C06.1 is the correct code.

2.18

The first organ listed in the block for malignant neoplasms of digestive organs is the <u>esophagus</u>.

Codes beginning with C15 are for malignant neoplasms of the esophagus. Look in your book and see that these are followed by stomach, small intestine, colon, rectosigmoid junction, rectum, anus and anal canal, liver and intrahepatic bile ducts, gallbladder, other and unspecified parts of biliary tract, and pancreas. There also are catch-all codes for other and ill-defined digestive organs.

2.19

The order of the glands in the malignant neoplasms of thyroid and other endocrine glands block is: <u>thyroid, adrenal and other</u>.

Malignant neoplasms of the thyroid gland are C73, *Malignant neoplasms of the adrenal gland* are C74 and *Malignant neoplasms of other endocrine glands and related structures* are C75.

2.20

The major code that comes after C75 is <u>C7A</u>.

Take Note! *Notice that the codes get a little different here. The next code after C75 is C7A Malignant neuroendocrine tumors and it is followed by codes beginning with C7B Secondary neuroendocrine tumors. The best rule to follow is not to assume that the codes will always be in logical order!*

2.21

You see a claim with a diagnosis code of C50.212. In which block is this included?

_____ In situ neoplasms   _____ Malignant neoplasms of breast

_____ Benign neuroendocrine   _____ Neoplasms of unspecified
    tumors   behavior

2.22

Let's look at **Block C43-C44** (Melanoma and other malignant neoplasms of skin).
Notice that the next major (unindented) code after C43 is C4A *Merkel cell carcinoma*.
How are the codes under C4A organized?

_____ By location (body part)   _____ By type of neoplasm

2.23

You see a claim for a benign neoplasm of the right ureter. Complete the code.

D30._____

2.24

You see a medical record for a patient who has a benign neoplasm of the
suprahyoid portion of the epiglottis. Complete the code.

D14._____

Take Note!
The Quick Quizzes are short exercises that refer
back to things you've already learned. The Chapter
Quizzes are longer than the Quick Quizzes. For these,
you can take your time, refer back to the exercises
and notes and think about the answers. You will find
all the answers in Appendix A.

2.21

The block for C50.212 is <u>Malignant neoplasms of breast</u>.

Look this up in your book. Notice that this six-character code is for malignant neoplasm of upper-inner quadrant of the left breast of a female. It's a perfect example of just how specific ICD-10 instructs you to be.

2.22

The codes under C4A are organized <u>by location (body part).</u>

The indented codes under C4A *Merkel cell carcinoma* are organized by body part. Some are further divided by unspecified, right or left and some are further divided by body part or unspecified.

2.23

The code is <u>D30.21</u> *Benign neoplasm of the right ureter*.

First, find D30. It is for benign neoplasm of urinary organs. Notice that D30 is further divided by organ: kidney, renal pelvis, ureter, bladder, urethra, other and finally a code for unspecified. Look for the organ on the claim, ureter. That's D30.2. Now find the right ureter and you have D30.21.

2.24

The code for a benign neoplasm of the suprahyoid portion of the epiglottis is <u>D14.1.</u>

Find D14 in your book. It is for benign neoplasms of the middle ear and the respiratory system. Notice that it is broken down into five sections. Look at the section for larynx and notice that beneath it is a note listing benign neoplasm of epiglottis (suprahyoid portion).

2.25

The patient has a malignant melanoma of the left shoulder. Complete the code.

C43._____

2.26

You see a claim for a malignant neoplasm of the sigmoid colon. Complete the code.
HINT: refer to the blocks at the beginning of the chapter.

C_____

2.27

A patient has a benign neoplasm of her left ovary. Complete the code.
HINT: consult the neoplasm table.

D_____

QUICK QUIZ *Answers in Appendix A*		
_____ 2.5 Primary malignant, middle lobe of lung	**A.** D26.1	
_____ 2.6 Carcinoma in situ of vulva	**B.** C34.2	
_____ 2.7 Benign, stem of brain	**C.** D33.1	
_____ 2.8 Benign, corpus of uterus	**D.** D07.1	
_____ 2.9 Basal cell carcinoma, scalp (skin)	**A.** C44.41	
_____ 2.10 Neoplasm of uncertain behavior, pancreas	**B.** C78.2	
_____ 2.11 Secondary malignant neoplasm, pleura	**C.** D37.8	
_____ 2.12 Benign neoplasm, bladder	**D.** D30.3	

2.25

The complete code for a *Malignant melanoma of the left shoulder* is <u>C43.62</u>.

First, look up C43 in your book. It is for *Malignant melanoma of the skin*. Notice that it is broken down by body part starting with lip, and then eyelid, followed by ear and so on. Find the shoulder. It is listed as upper limb, including shoulder, C43.6. Now find the code for the left side. It's C43.62.

2.26

The complete code for a *Malignant neoplasm of the sigmoid colon* is <u>C18.7</u>.

Did you go to the block for digestive organs (**C15-C26**)? As you look through this section you see that it is organized by body part: esophagus, stomach, small intestine and then colon (C18). Next, find the part of the colon – sigmoid, code C18.7.

2.27

The complete code for a *Benign neoplasm of the left ovary* is <u>D27.1</u>.

The quickest way to find this code is to use the neoplasm table. Look up the site of the neoplasm (ovary). As you scan across the table, find the column for benign, code D27. Now, find D27 in the tabular list and look for the left ovary. It's code D27.1.

QUICK QUIZ *Answers in Appendix A*

_____ 2.13 In situ	*A.*	Tissue
_____ 2.14 -plasm	*B.*	In position; localized
_____ 2.15 hist	*C.*	Study of
_____ 2.16 -ology	*D.*	Form

Chapter Quiz (Answers in Appendix A)

Match the definition to the word. Some of the Greek and Latin terms from this chapter are bold.

_____ 2.1	Cancerous	A. Neoplasm
_____ 2.2	The study of tissues or cells	B. Benign
_____ 2.3	Tumor or growth	C. Lymph**oma**
_____ 2.4	Cancer that develops in mesothelium	D. Morph**ology**
_____ 2.5	Non-cancerous	E. Malignant
_____ 2.6	Dark tumor on skin	F. Mesotheli**oma**
_____ 2.7	Localized neoplasm	G. Melan**oma**
_____ 2.8	Lymphatic system cancer	H. In situ
_____ 2.9	The study of the shape or form of cells	I. Carcin**oma**
_____ 2.10	Cancerous tumor	J. Hist**ology**

Match the description to the code.

_____ 2.11	Malignant neoplasm of upper gum	A. D33.0
_____ 2.12	Hepatosplenic T-cell lymphoma	B. C37
_____ 2.13	Liver cell carcinoma	C. C08.1
_____ 2.14	Benign neoplasm of cecum	D. D03.0
_____ 2.15	Benign neoplasm of brain, supratentorial	E. C45.0
_____ 2.16	Melanoma in situ of lip	F. C86.1
_____ 2.17	Malignant neoplasm of sublingual gland	G. D12.0
_____ 2.18	Malignant neoplasm of thymus	H. C03.0
_____ 2.19	Benign neoplasm of right retina	I. C22.0
_____ 2.20	Mesothelioma of pleura	J. D31.21

Match the code to the block title the code is in.

_____ 2.21 C71.3	A. Malignant neoplasms of lip, oral cavity and pharynx
_____ 2.22 D06.0	B. Malignant neoplasms of digestive organs
_____ 2.23 C7B.02	C. Malignant neoplasms of respiratory and intrathoracic organs
_____ 2.24 C62.11	D. Malignant neoplasms of bone and articular cartilage
_____ 2.25 C7A.023	E. Melanoma and other malignant neoplasms of skin
_____ 2.26 D47.1	F. Malignant neoplasms of mesothelial and soft tissue
_____ 2.27 C76.51	G. Malignant neoplasms of breast
_____ 2.28 D24.1	H. Malignant neoplasms of female genital organs
_____ 2.29 C40.22	I. Malignant neoplasms of male genital organs
_____ 2.30 C75.1	J. Malignant neoplasms of urinary tract
_____ 2.31 C09.9	K. Malignant neoplasms of eye, brain and other parts of central nervous system
_____ 2.32 C66.1	L. Malignant neoplasms of thyroid and other endocrine glands
_____ 2.33 C44.212	M. Malignant neuroendocrine tumors
_____ 2.34 C34.31	N. Secondary neuroendocrine tumors
_____ 2.35 C50.312	O. Malignant neoplasms of ill-defined, other secondary and unspecified sites
_____ 2.36 D3A.024	P. Malignant neoplasms of lymphoid, hematopoietic and related tissue
_____ 2.37 C18.4	Q. In situ neoplasms
_____ 2.38 C57.01	R. Benign neoplasms, except benign neuroendocrine tumors
_____ 2.39 C81.37	S. Benign neuroendocrine tumors
_____ 2.40 C47.11	T. Neoplasms of uncertain behavior, polycythemia vera and myelodysplastic syndromes

3

Diseases of the Blood and Blood-forming Organs and Certain Disorders Involving the Immune Mechanism

Chapter 3 in the ICD-10 book has a very long name and can sound intimidating. Don't worry, it's a small chapter of just seven blocks and by the time you finish this chapter, you'll have a good grasp of what it covers. Let's take a look.

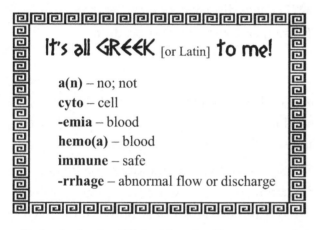

It's all GREEK [or Latin] to me!

a(n) – no; not
cyto – cell
-emia – blood
hemo(a) – blood
immune – safe
-rrhage – abnormal flow or discharge

The first three blocks cover types of anemias. Anemia is a condition in which the blood doesn't have enough red blood cells. The prefix *an-* comes from the Greek and means no or not. The suffix *-emia* also comes from Greek and means blood. Red blood cells carry oxygen to the cells in the body. White blood cells are part of the immune system. They help the body fight off disease.

A type of white blood cell responsible for the body's protection against infection is called a neutrophil cell. An abnormally low number of neutrophil cells in the blood is called neutropenia. The suffix *-penia* comes from the Greek word meaning lack.

The medical term for an abnormal flow or discharge of blood is hemorrhage. Hemorrhage has two word parts: *hemo-* from the Greek word meaning blood, and *-rrhage* from the Greek word meaning an abnormal flow or discharge. You can see an example of it being used in a diagnosis by looking at D78.0 *Intraoperative hemorrhage and hematoma of the spleen complicating a procedure.*

Hematoma is a collection of blood outside of a blood vessel. A hematoma is caused by a break in a blood vessel. Hematoma also has two word parts: *hema-* which means blood and *-oma* which means a tumor or swelling. (The t in the middle is added to make it easier to pronounce.)

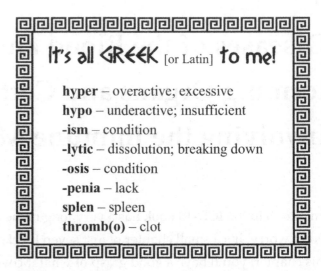

It's all GREEK [or Latin] to me!

hyper – overactive; excessive
hypo – underactive; insufficient
-ism – condition
-lytic – dissolution; breaking down
-osis – condition
-penia – lack
splen – spleen
thromb(o) – clot

The spleen is an organ that serves as a blood filter. One of its functions is to remove old red blood cells. Disorders of the spleen are found in **Block D70-D77** (Other disorders of blood and blood-forming organs) and in **Block D78** (Intraoperative and postprocedural complications of the spleen).

Let's consider the terms hyposplenism and hypersplenism. Find code D73.0 *Hyposplenism* in your code book. Then look at the next code, D73.1 *Hypersplenism*. What's the difference in these two terms? The secret is in the prefixes: *hypo-* and *hyper-*. *Hypo-* comes from the Greek word meaning under, reduced or smaller. *Hyper-* comes from the Greek word meaning over, excess, or big. Splenism refers to the functioning of the spleen. Therefore, hyposplenism is a condition in which the spleen is not working as well as it should and hypersplenism is a condition in which the spleen is working in overdrive.

Knowing the basic root words will allow you to see exceptionally long and complicated medical terms for the first time and get a very good idea what it means. For example, find **Block D65-D69** and look at D69.4 and D69.5 thrombocytopenia. This is a large word but it is easy to understand when you break it into the root parts. *Thrombo-* comes from the Greek word for clot, *cyto-* comes from the Greek word meaning cell (in this case the platelets) and *-penia*, as you know, comes from the Greek word meaning lack. So, you know that thrombocytopenia is a condition involving a deficiency of platelets (cells that cause clotting) in the blood.

Another basic medical suffix you'll come across throughout the ICD-10 is *-osis*. It comes from Greek and indicates a condition. For example, sarcoidosis (code D86) is a condition in which numerous lesions form.

Here's one more term that you can dissect and figure out the meaning. The second block of codes **D55-D59** is for hemolytic anemias. You already know *hemo-* means blood. The suffix *-lytic* comes from the Greek word for dissolution or breaking down. Therefore, hemolytic means the breaking down of red blood cells.

Practice the codes in Chapter 3 by answering these questions.

3.1

Pedro has a hemorrhage, an abnormal discharge or flow of blood. It is due to acquired hemophilia. Go to D68 and decide which complete code best describes this condition?

_____ D68.318   _____ D68.311   _____ D68.32

3.2

Dr. Livingston's first patient this morning has sickle cell anemia. Which code describes this condition?

_____ D51.0   _____ D69.49   _____ D57.1

3.3

Juanita has been diagnosed with thrombocytopenia which in her case is hereditary. Which is the code for this condition?

_____ D50.0   _____ D69.42   _____ D57.2

QUICK QUIZ *Answers in Appendix A*

_____ 3.1 Non-cancerous		*A.* Melan
_____ 3.2 New		*B.* -oma
_____ 3.3 Tumor; swelling		*C.* Neo
_____ 3.4 Dark		*D.* Benign

3.1

<u>D68.311</u> is the code for acquired hemophilia.

Hemo- means blood. *-rrhage* means an abnormal flow or discharge. Look at **Block D65-D69** (Coagulation defects, purpura and other hemorrhagic conditions) in your ICD-10 book. You will see several codes concerning hemorrhaging.

3.2

Sickle-cell disorder is a condition in which the patient has abnormal red blood cells that are crescent, or sickle, shaped. Sickle-cell disorders begin with code D57. Therefore, <u>D57.1</u> is the best choice.

Sickle-cell anemia is the most commonly known sickle-cell disorder.

3.3

The correct code is <u>D69.42</u> *Congenital and hereditary thrombocytopenia purpura.*

Thrombocytopenia is made up of three word parts: *thrombo-* comes from the Greek word for clot, *cyto-* means cell (referring to the platelets) and *-penia* meaning lack.

There's a code for THAT??

Was it a frog or a toad? Was it venomous or non-venomous? But wait: there's more! Was the harmful contact with this amphibian accidental or intentional? What if it actually turns into a prince? Codes for contact with venomous frogs and toads are found in Chapter 19 while codes for non-venomous ones are in Chapter 20. Just kidding about the prince. Note that there are codes for other amphibians, too.

3.4

Dr. Livingston's next patient this morning has anemia. She doesn't have enough iron in her blood cells. What is one of the codes for this condition?

_____ D86.1   _____ D50.8

_____ D59.0   _____ D70.4

3.5

Dr. Livingston's next patient has neutropenia, a condition in which the blood has an abnormally small number of a particular type of white blood cell called neutrophil cells. Which code is for this condition?

_____ D86.1   _____ D50.8

_____ D59.0   _____ D70.4

3.6

The next patient has a condition called drug-induced autoimmune hemolytic anemia. Which code describes this condition?

_____ D86.1   _____ D50.8

_____ D59.0   _____ D70.4

3.7

Another patient comes to see Dr. Livingston about numerous lesions, which the doctor has diagnosed as sarcoidosis of the lymph nodes. Which code is this?

_____ D86.1   _____ D50.8

_____ D59.0   _____ D70.4

3.8

Mary Sue's claim indicates a blood condition coded D72.819. Look up the code and name the type of blood cells.

_____ Red blood cells   _____ White blood cells

3.4

<u>D50.8</u> *Other iron deficiency anemias* is the correct code.

Anemia has many codes. ICD-10 requires you to be specific in selecting the most appropriate one.

3.5

The code for this patient is <u>D70.4</u> *Cyclic neutropenia*

The suffix *-penia* means lack. Neutrophil cells are a type of white blood cell responsible for the body's protection against infection. Combine neutro with *-penia* and you get the term neutropenia.

3.6

The correct answer is <u>D59.0</u>.

Check out the block of codes **D55-D59** (Hemolytic anemias). Category D59 is for acquired hemolytic anemia. Remember: *hemo-* = blood; *-lytic* = breaking down.

3.7

The correct code is <u>D86.1</u>.

Category D86 is for sarcoidosis. Indented codes below that further define areas of the body. That is where you find lymph nodes. Remember: *-osis* = condition.

3.8

The answer is <u>white blood cells</u>, part of the immune system that fights disease.

Red blood cells are responsible for carrying oxygen to the cells of the body.

QUICK QUIZ Answers in Appendix A

_____ 3.5 NOS meaning	**A.** Seven
_____ 3.6 The minimum number of characters in a code	**B.** Unspecified
_____ 3.7 Used as a placeholder character	**C.** Three
_____ 3.8 The maximum number of characters in a code	**D.** The letter X

3.9

Billy has a condition involving his spleen. Which of these categories is for diseases
of the spleen?

_____ D71   _____ D72
_____ D73   _____ D74

3.10

One of Dr. Livingston's patients has a condition in which the spleen is working
overtime, called hypersplenism. What is the code for this condition?

_____ D73.1   _____ D73.0

3.11

Dr. Livingston has another patient who has the opposite problem, hyposplenism.
What is the code for this condition?

_____ D73.1   _____ D73.0

3.12

Look at the blocks at the beginning of this chapter. Under what block does D57.21
fall?

_____ Nutritional anemias
_____ Hemolytic anemias
_____ Aplastic and other anemias
_____ Coagulation defects

3.13

You see a medical record with a diagnosis of selective deficiency of
immunoglobulin M [IgM]. Complete the code.

D80._____

62   Chapter 3

3.9

<u>D73</u> is for diseases of the spleen. The spleen is involved in blood formation. It is also responsible for filtering the blood and removing old blood cells.

3.10

Hypersplenism is a condition in which the spleen removes excessive amounts of blood cells from circulation. Code <u>D73.1</u> is for *Hypersplenism*.

Hyper- means excess. In this condition, hypersplenism, the spleen is removing more blood cells than it should.

3.11

Hyposplenism is a condition in which the spleen is functioning at a lower level than it should. Find code <u>D73.0</u> *Hyposplenism*.

Hypo- means reduced.

Another prefix to know is *a-*, which means not. It is used to indicate something is not there or not functioning at all. In this case, asplenia indicates a condition worse than hyposplenism. In asplenia the spleen is not working at all or is just barely working.

3.12

D57.21 falls under the block: <u>Hemolytic anemias</u>.

Nutritional anemias are covered in **Block D50-D53**; Hemolytic anemias are found in **Block D55-D59**; Aplastic and other anemias are found in **Block D60-D64**; Coagulation defects are covered in **Block D65-D69**.

3.13

<u>D80.4</u> is the code for *Selective deficiency of immunoglobulin M [IgM]*.

Look at the indented codes under D80. There are several for selective deficiency of immunoglobulin. You'll see that the code specifically for immunoglobulin M [IgM] is D80.4.

ICD-10-CM Quick Learn©

This chapter contains some very important notes.

Pay special attention to the notes as you answer the following questions.

3.14

You see a claim with two codes: D61.810 and D61.1. Can these two codes be used at the same time? How do you know?

_____ Yes   _____ No

3.15

Is sarcoidosis included in the code range D80-D89?

_____ Yes   _____ No

3.16

Is it ok to use one of the D56 codes with D57.411? Why or why not?

_____ Yes   _____ No

3.17

Is it ok to code N17.0 with D59.3? Why or why not?

_____ Yes   _____ No

3.18

You see a claim that has both D73.1 and D73.81 on the claim. Is it coded correctly?

_____ Yes   _____ No

QUICK QUIZ *Answers in Appendix A*

_____ 3.9 Respiratory system   *A.* Codes begin with N

_____ 3.10 Symptoms and signs   *B.* Codes begin with R

_____ 3.11 Eye and adnexa   *C.* Codes begin with J

_____ 3.12 Genitourinary system   *D.* Codes begin with H

3.14

Yes, codes D61.810 and D61.1 can be used at the same time.

Just below code D61.810 is an **Excludes2** note. **Excludes2** notes mean that it is ok to use both codes on the same claim.

3.15

Yes, sarcoidosis is included in the range D80-D89.

Read the **Includes** note at the beginning of the block entitled Certain disorders involving the immune mechanism. It appears just before code D80. Sarcoidosis is one of the listed diagnoses, D86.

3.16

No, it is not ok to use one of the D56 codes with D57.411.

Why not? The **Excludes1** note after D56 says you cannot use a D56 code with any sickle-cell thalassemia code: D57.4-.

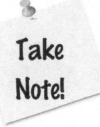

Remember: **Excludes1** = NOT.

Excludes1 notes mean that the two conditions indicated cannot be coded at the same time.

3.17

Yes, it is ok to code N17.0 with D59.3.

How do you know? Because the note after code D59.3 specifically says to code also any associated N17 codes if applicable.

3.18

No, it is not ok to code both D73.1 and D73.81 on the same claim.

Why not? There is an **Excludes1** note after D73.1 that lists D73.81. This note tells you these two codes should not be used together.

Chapter Quiz (Answers in Appendix A)

Using your knowledge of Greek and Latin root words, match the definition to the term. Some of the Greek and Latin terms from this chapter are bold.

_____ 3.1	Abnormal discharge of blood	A. Hemo**rrhage**
_____ 3.2	The spleen is removing too many cells	B. -ism
_____ 3.3	Term meaning lack	C. Neutro**penia**
_____ 3.4	Term meaning dissolution	D. Sarcoid**osis**
_____ 3.5	Term meaning condition	E. -emia
_____ 3.6	Not enough platelets in the blood	F. An**emia**
_____ 3.7	Term meaning blood	G. Hypo**splen**ism
_____ 3.8	Numerous lesions throughout the body	H. Thrombo**cyto**penia
_____ 3.9	Not enough red blood cells	I. Hyper**splen**ism
_____ 3.10	The spleen is not functioning too well	J. Hemo**lytic**
_____ 3.11	Not enough neutrophil cells	K. A**splen**ia
_____ 3.12	The spleen is not functioning at all	L. -penia
_____ 3.13	Red blood cells are breaking down	M. -lytic

Match the code to the block title the code is in.

_____ 3.14	D61.810	A. Nutritional anemias
_____ 3.15	D78.21	B. Hemolytic anemias
_____ 3.16	D52.0	C. Aplastic and other anemias and other bone marrow failure syndromes
_____ 3.17	D69.0	D. Coagulation defects, purpura and other hemorrhagic conditions
_____ 3.18	D86.3	E. Other disorders of blood and blood forming organs
_____ 3.19	D57.411	F. Interoperative and postprocedural complications of the spleen
_____ 3.20	D70.0	G. Certain disorders involving the immune mechanism

Match the items on the left with the corresponding item on the right.

_____ 3.21	NOS meaning	A. Etiology
_____ 3.22	Example of content in a category	B. **Includes** note
_____ 3.23	Underlying condition coded first	C. **Excludes1** note
_____ 3.24	Never use codes at the same time	D. **Excludes2** note
_____ 3.25	The minimum characters in a code	E. Unspecified
_____ 3.26	The maximum characters in a code	F. Seven
_____ 3.27	Used as a placeholder character	G. Three
_____ 3.28	You must use a different code, but can be coded at the same time	H. The letter X

Match the chapter to the first letter(s) of the code.

_____ 3.29	Digestive system	C or D
_____ 3.30	Blood and blood forming organs	D
_____ 3.31	Endocrine, nutritional and metabolic diseases	E
_____ 3.32	Skin and subcutaneous tissue	G
_____ 3.33	Congenital malformations, deformations and chromosomal abnormalities	H
		I
_____ 3.34	Factors influencing health status	K
_____ 3.35	Ear and mastoid process	L
_____ 3.36	Circulatory system	Q
_____ 3.37	Nervous system	R
_____ 3.38	External causes of morbidity	V, W, X or Y
_____ 3.39	Symptoms, signs and abnormal clinical and laboratory findings, NEC	Z
_____ 3.40	Neoplasms	

4

Endocrine, Nutritional and Metabolic Diseases

The endocrine glands secrete hormones directly into the bloodstream rather than through ducts. The major endocrine glands are: The **pituitary gland,** also called the master gland (located at the base of the brain), the **thyroid gland** (located in the neck), the **parathyroid glands** (located close to the thyroid), the **pineal gland** (located near the center of the brain), the **adrenal glands** (located on top of the kidneys), the **thymus** (located in the chest), the **gonads** (ovaries in females, testicles in males) and the **pancreas** (located behind the stomach).

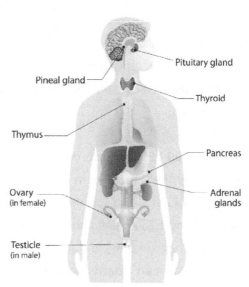

Let's look at some of the codes, blocks, terminology, prefixes, suffixes and root words found in Chapter 4.

Find code E06 *Thyroiditis*. Thyroiditis is the inflammation of the thyroid. If you remember the prefixes *hypo-* and *hyper-*, you can deduce what hyperthyroidism and hypothyroidism mean. Hyperthyroidism is an overactive thyroid and hypothyroidism is an underactive thyroid. You will find thyroiditis in **Block E00-E07** (Disorders of the thyroid gland).

Another condition that affects the thyroid is goiter, an enlargement of the thyroid. It can have many causes, so ICD-10 provides several codes for you to select from, for example code E01.0 *Iodine-deficiency related diffuse (endemic) goiter*.

Diabetes occurs when the body does not produce enough insulin. Look at the list of blocks at the beginning of this chapter. Diabetes mellitus has its own block: **E08-E13**. If you look through this block in the ICD-10 you will see hundreds of codes for diabetes.

It's all GREEK [or Latin] **to me!**

-itis – inflammation
pancrea – pancreas
para – alongside of
poly – many

Block E15-E16 (Other disorders of glucose regulation and pancreatic internal secretion) has only two codes: E15 *Nondiabetic hypoglycemic coma* and E16 *Other disorders of pancreatic internal secretion*. E16 has several indented codes beneath it.

Look in **Block E20-E35** (Disorders of other endocrine glands) and some of the diagnoses you will see may seem difficult to translate but they are almost all just combinations of Greek and Latin roots. Some examples: E22 *Hyperfunction of pituitary gland* and E23 *Hypofunction and other disorders of the pituitary gland*. We learned both *hyper-* (excess) and *hypo-* (reduced) in Chapter 3. In the chart above you see that poly means many. So E31 *Polyglandular dysfunction* means it involves more than one gland.

Block E36 (Intraoperative complications of endocrine system) contains codes for problems arising during an operation. As you progress through the book you will see that several chapters have a block similar to this one.

Find **Block E65-E68** (Overweight, obesity and other hyperalimentation). You know what *hyper-* means. Alimentation is from the Latin for nourishment or food.

Metabolic (from Greek for change) is an important term that you will see throughout this chapter and in other chapters of the ICD-10. It refers to the biochemical processes that occur in a living organism. **Block E70-E88** is for metabolic disorders.

The last block in this chapter is **E89** (Postprocedural endocrine and metabolic complications and disorders, not elsewhere classified). Many chapters have codes for disorders occurring after a medical procedure that cannot be classified elsewhere.

Now, practice looking up some codes.

4.1

Code E16 involves what organ.

_____ Pancreas   _____ Stomach   _____ Gall bladder

4.2

Which gland, located in the neck, is the focus of the first block of codes?

_____ Thyroid gland   _____ Thymus gland   _____ Gonads

4.3

Which of these codes are indented beneath "Other hyperalimentation?"

_____ E67.0 and E67.3   _____ E64.3 and E64.8   _____ E61.5 and E61.8

4.4

Block E40-E46 covers which condition(s)?

_____ Diabetes mellitus   _____ Metabolic disorder
_____ Malnutrition   _____ Other nutritional deficiencies

4.1

The correct answer is the <u>pancreas</u>.

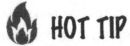

HOT TIP

There are a few codes for pancreas in this chapter.
But codes for the pancreas are also listed in the
chapter for diseases of the digestive system. If you
look up pancreas in the alphabetical index, you'll
find the instruction: "See condition." You should
always first search the index by condition.

4.2

The correct answer is <u>the thyroid gland</u>.

Block E00-E07 covers disorders of the thyroid gland.

4.3

<u>E67.0 and E67.3</u> are indented beneath E67 *Other hyperalimentation.*

4.4

Block E40-E46 is for <u>malnutrition</u>.

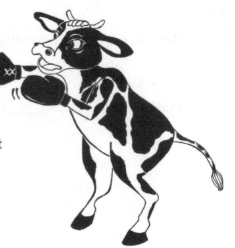

There's a code for THAT??

Injury by cow? ICD-10 requires details!
Was the patient bitten, struck or perhaps it
was some other kind of contact? Check
category W55.2 for code choices.

4.5

Riley has a condition involving one of his endocrine glands. His diagnosis is E32.0. Which gland is it?

_____ The thyroid gland   _____ The thymus gland   _____ The gonads

4.6

Codes E28 and E29 refer to what gland(s)?

_____ The thyroid gland   _____ The thymus gland   _____ The gonads

4.7

Bill's doctor has diagnosed a condition relating to his pituitary gland. Which code refers to this gland?

_____ E34.8   _____ E20.0
_____ E22.8   _____ E27.1

4.8

Reba has an endocrine condition involving the gland located near the center of her brain, the pineal gland. Which code refers to this gland?

_____ E34.8   _____ E20.0
_____ E22.8   _____ E27.1

QUICK QUIZ *Answers in Appendix A*

_____ 4.1	Underlying condition coded first	**A. Excludes1** note
_____ 4.2	Examples of content in a category	**B. Includes** note
_____ 4.3	Codes should not be used at the same time	**C.** Etiology/manifestation
_____ 4.4	You must use a different code, but can be used at the same time	**D. Excludes2** note

4.5

The correct answer is <u>the thymus gland</u>. E32.0 indicates that Riley has persistent hyperplasia of the thymus.

4.6

E28 and E29 refer to <u>the gonads</u>.

The gonads in females are called the ovaries. They produce estrogens.

In males, the gonads are the testes. They produce testosterone.

4.7

<u>E22.8</u> refers to the pituitary gland.

It is called the master gland because it controls many bodily functions including the functioning of other glands. The pituitary gland has two lobes: anterior pituitary and posterior pituitary.

4.8

<u>E34.8</u> is for the pineal gland.

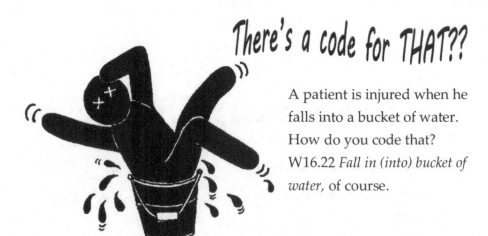

There's a code for THAT??

A patient is injured when he falls into a bucket of water. How do you code that? W16.22 *Fall in (into) bucket of water*, of course.

4.9

John has idiopathic hypoparathyroidism. Which code applies to his condition?

_____ E34.8   _____ E20.0
_____ E22.8   _____ E27.1

4.10

Javier has primary adrenocortical insufficiency, a condition which affects the adrenal gland. Which code is used for this diagnosis?

_____ E34.8   _____ E20.0
_____ E22.8   _____ E27.1

4.11

Which code is for hypothyroidism, the condition of insufficient or below normal thyroid hormone?

_____ E05   _____ E03.9
_____ E04.2   _____ E06.0

4.12

A patient comes to the doctor with thyroiditis, inflammation of the thyroid. Which of the following codes applies?

_____ E05   _____ E03.9
_____ E04.2   _____ E06.0

4.13

Another patient presents at the doctor's office with a condition in which there is an overproduction of the thyroid hormone. The diagnosis is hyperthyroidism. Which code applies?

_____ E05   _____ E03.9
_____ E04.2   _____ E06.0

4.9

E20.0 is the code for idiopathic hypoparathyroidism.

Codes E20 and E21 are for the parathyroid gland.

4.10

E27.1 is the code for primary adrenocortical insufficiency.

The adrenal glands are best known for producing **adrenal**ine, the hormone that allows you to spring into action in a stressful situation, but they produce other essential hormones. Note that E27 has indented codes regarding the type of condition.

4.11

Code E03.9 *Hypothyroidism, unspecified* is one of the codes used when the production of the thyroid hormone is below normal.

Hypo- is a prefix that means insufficient or below.

4.12

E06.0 is the correct answer. Thyroiditis is the inflammation or swelling of the thyroid.

Remember that the suffix *-itis* indicates inflammation. Did you notice the many codes indented beneath E06 which specify several causes and types of thyroiditis?

4.13

E05 is for hyperthyroidism. Look up E05 in the ICD-10 and notice all the indented codes which indicate the types of hyperthyroidism. Remember, in coding you must select the most detailed code.

Hyper- means excessive. The ICD-10 lists hyperthyroidism as thyrotoxicosis because these terms are often used interchangeably.

4.14

Minerva has a nontoxic multinodular goiter in the thyroid gland. Which of these codes is it?

_____ E05   _____ E03.9

_____ E04.2   _____ E06.0

4.15

Diabetes mellitus is a result of inadequate production of insulin or inadequate sensitivity to, or even resistance to, insulin. Which code applies to this diagnosis?

_____ E08.311   _____ E66.09

_____ E70.40   _____ E31.8

4.16

Obesity is a condition in which there is an excessive amount of fat on the body. Which code applies to this condition?

_____ E08.311   _____ E66.09

_____ E70.40   _____ E31.8

4.17

A patient comes to the doctor's office with a condition involving several of the endocrine glands. Which code would be most appropriate?

_____ E08.311   _____ E66.09

_____ E70.40   _____ E31.8

4.18

Which code involves metabolism?

_____ E08.311   _____ E66.09

_____ E70.40   _____ E31.8

4.14

E04.2 is one of the goiter codes.

4.15

E08.311 is the correct answer.

Diabetes mellitus has its own block in the ICD-10: **E08-E13**.

4.16

E66.09 is one of the obesity codes.

Obesity is in **Block E65-E68** (Overweight, obesity and other hyperalimentation).

4.17

The codes indented beneath E31 are all for polyglandular dysfunctions. A polyglandular dysfunction involves several of the endocrine glands.

Poly- is a prefix that means many. Polyglandular means many glands.

4.18

E70.40 is the correct answer. In the ICD-10 you will see that the block of codes for metabolic disorders is **E70-E88**.

Metabolic refers to the range of biochemical processes that a living organism uses to stay alive. For example, the process of making energy from the food you eat.

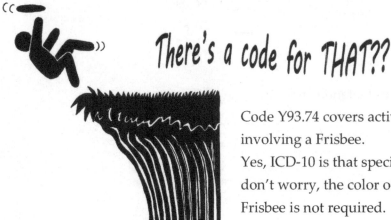

There's a code for THAT??

Code Y93.74 covers activities involving a Frisbee.
Yes, ICD-10 is that specific! But, don't worry, the color of the Frisbee is not required.

4.19

Look at the list of blocks contained in this chapter. Is diabetes one of the blocks?

_____ Yes _____ No

4.20

Is obesity one of the blocks?

_____ Yes _____ No

4.21

Is metabolic disorders one of the blocks?

_____ Yes _____ No

4.22

Which of the following codes are for diabetes mellitus?

_____ E08 _____ E09
_____ E10 _____ E11
_____ E12 _____ E13
_____ None of these _____ All of these

4.23

The doctor has diagnosed a patient with iodine deficiency (E00.1) which has caused some moderate intellectual deficiencies. This seems to be two issues, would you use two codes for this?

_____ Yes _____ No

4.24

You see a claim with two diagnosis codes: P35.0 and E08.01. Which way should the codes be ordered? Hint: read the **"Code first"** note with E08.

_____ E08.01 and then P35.0 _____ P35.0 and then E08.01

4.19

Yes, diabetes is one of the blocks in this chapter.

Diabetes mellitus is the block of codes **E08-E13**.

4.20

Yes, obesity is one of the blocks in this chapter.

Codes **E65-E68** cover overweight, obesity and other hyperalimentation.

4.21

Yes, metabolic disorders are covered in the block of codes **E70-E88**.

4.22

All of these codes are for diabetes mellitus.

The codes for diabetes mellitus are **E08-E13**.

4.23

Yes, the **"Use additional code"** note under E00 instructs you to use an additional code (F70-F79) to identify associated intellectual disabilities.

In this case, you will find moderate intellectual deficiencies under F71.

4.24

The correct way to order these two codes is P35.0 and then E08.01.

The **"Code first"** note after E08 instructs you to enter the underlying condition first. P35.0 is listed as an underlying condition for E08.

QUICK QUIZ *Answers in Appendix A*

_____ 4.5 Originating in the perinatal period	**A.** Codes begin with O
_____ 4.6 Pregnancy and childbirth	**B.** Codes begin with G
_____ 4.7 Digestive system	**C.** Codes begin with P
_____ 4.8 Nervous system	**D.** Codes begin with K

4.25

You see a claim with two diagnosis codes: H42 and E72.03. Which way should the codes be ordered?

_____ E72.03 and then H42   _____ H42 and then E72.03

4.26

One of Dr. Livingston's patients has a diagnosis of familial hypophosphatemia. What are the last two digits of this code?

E83._____

4.27

Look under **Block E50-E64** (Other nutritional deficiencies) and find the first part of the code for vitamin A deficiency with night blindness.

_____.5

4.28

The doctor tells her patient that he has type 2 diabetes mellitus with diabetic neuropathic arthropathy. Complete the code for this diagnosis.

E11._____

4.29

You see a claim that has both E06.1 and E06.3 used together. Which type of note indicates that this is coded incorrectly?

_____ **Excludes1**   _____ **Excludes2**
_____ **"Use additional code"**   _____ **"Code first"**

4.25

The correct order for these codes is <u>E72.03 and then H42</u>.

This is explained in the "**Use additional code**" note following code E72.03.

4.26

The last two digits are <u>.31</u>. The complete code for familial hypophosphatemia is E83.31.

E83 is a perfect example of the necessity to read all notes. Sometimes the notes you need are listed with the higher category, but notes can also show up in individual codes, the category, the block and the chapter. Pay attention to all of them.

4.27

The first part of the code for vitamin A deficiency with night blindness is <u>E50.</u>

The complete code is E50.5.

4.28

The complete code for *Type 2 diabetes mellitus with diabetic neuropathic arthropathy* is <u>E11.610</u>.

The codes that begin with E11 are for type 2 diabetes mellitus. As you look at the indented codes you will see they are divided by complication. E11.6 is for other specified complications, E11.61 is for diabetic arthropathy, and finally, E11.610 is for diabetic neuropathic arthropathy.

4.29

The note is <u>**Excludes1**</u>.

Find E06.1 in your book. The **Excludes1** note specifically mentions E06.3 instructing you not to use these codes together.

Chapter Quiz (Answers in Appendix A)

Let's review some Greek and Latin terms and definitions that we covered in the first four chapters. Match the definition to the word part.

_____ 4.1	Tumor; swelling	A. cyto
_____ 4.2	Tissue	B. hyper
_____ 4.3	Condition	C. -itis
_____ 4.4	Cell	D. safe
_____ 4.5	Abnormal flow or discharge	E. poly
_____ 4.6	Overactive; excessive	F. -oma
_____ 4.7	Dark	G. -lytic
_____ 4.8	Lack	H. hist
_____ 4.9	Inflammation	I. -ism
_____ 4.10	Alongside of	J. morph
_____ 4.11	Many	K. melan
_____ 4.12	Dissolution; breaking down	L. -osis
_____ 4.13	Underactive; insufficient	M. a(n)
_____ 4.14	Study of	N. hypo
_____ 4.15	Condition	O. -emia
_____ 4.16	Blood	P. para
_____ 4.17	No; not	Q. -rrhage
_____ 4.18	Non-cancerous	R. -penia
_____ 4.19	Immune	S. -ology
_____ 4.20	Form; shape	T. benign

Match the code to the block title the code is in.

_____ 4.21	E16.1	A.	Disorders of thyroid gland
_____ 4.22	E11.22	B.	Diabetes mellitus
_____ 4.23	E44.1	C.	Other disorders of glucose regulation and pancreatic internal secretion
_____ 4.24	E89.3	D.	Disorders of other endocrine glands
_____ 4.25	E06.0	E.	Interoperative complications of endocrine system
_____ 4.26	E31.1	F.	Malnutrition
_____ 4.27	E55.0	G.	Other nutritional deficiencies
_____ 4.28	E36.01	H.	Overweight, obesity and other hyperalimentation
_____ 4.29	E66.2	I.	Metabolic disorders
_____ 4.30	E84.19	J.	Postprocedural endocrine and metabolic complications and disorders, not elsewhere classified

Match the diagnosis description to the code.

_____ 4.31	Other hypoglycemia	A.	E11.9
_____ 4.32	Sequela of rickets	B.	E23.0
_____ 4.33	Nontoxic diffuse goiter	C.	E87.6
_____ 4.34	Hypopituitarism	D.	E21.0
_____ 4.35	Wet beriberi	E.	E51.12
_____ 4.36	Type 2 diabetes without complications	F.	E72.53
_____ 4.37	Primary hyperoxaluria	G.	E04.0
_____ 4.38	Abscess of thymus	H.	E16.1
_____ 4.39	Primary hyperparathyroidism	I.	E64.3
_____ 4.40	Hypokalemia	J.	E32.1

5

Mental, Behavioral and Neurodevelopmental Disorders

The codes in Chapter 5 begin with F. Join us as we take a tour of this chapter. Let's start at the top: **F01-F09**. The first code, F01, is for vascular dementia. Dementia is a widespread disease involving loss of the ability to think.

The second block is **F10-F19** (Mental and behavioral disorders due to psychoactive substance use). This block includes alcohol and drug abuse codes. The term psychoactive is made of two word parts. *Psych-* comes from the Greek word for mind. So psychoactive means to act on the mind, or to alter perception or mood.

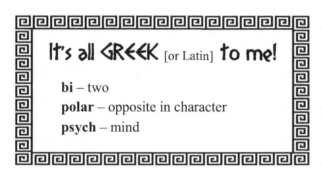

It's all GREEK [or Latin] to me!

bi – two
polar – opposite in character
psych – mind

The codes in this block are broken down by the type of substance abused. For example, F10 is for alcohol, F11 is opioids, F12 is cannabis, F13 is sedative, hypnotic, or anxiolytic related disorders.

F20-F29 (Schizophrenia, schizotypal, delusional, and other non-mood psychotic disorders) is the next block. You know that *psych-* means mind and *-osis* comes from Greek meaning an abnormal condition or disease. Psychosis means an abnormal condition of the mind with loss of contact with reality.

Block F30-F39 is for mood [affective] disorders. Affective refers to moods or feelings. For example, code F30 is for manic episode, F31 is for bipolar disorder, and F32 is for depressive episode. Bipolar disorder indicates that the patient has both manic and depressive episodes.

The next block is **F40-F48** (Anxiety, dissociative, stress-related, somatoform and other nonpsychotic mental disorders). Dissociative indicates a disruption of memory, perception or awareness. There are specific codes for different types of dissociative disorders. F44 is for dissociative and conversion disorders. Now look at F45. *Soma-*

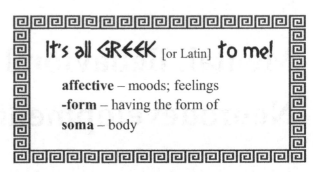

It's all GREEK [or Latin] to me!

affective – moods; feelings
-form – having the form of
soma – body

comes from the Greek word for body and *-form* is Latin for "having the form of." Somatoform is a condition that has the form of a bodily disease but there is no disease.

Block F50-F59 is for behavioral syndromes associated with physiological disturbances and physical factors. Examples are F50 which is eating disorders, F51 for sleep disorders, and F52 which is sexual dysfunction.

Block F60-F69 is for disorders of adult personality and behavior. F60, for example has indented codes including paranoid personality disorder and antisocial personality disorder. It also includes impulsive disorders such as pathological gambling and pyromania.

Take Note!

There are some important notes at the beginning of Block F70-F79 (Intellectual disabilities). **"Code first"** informs you to code any associated physical or development disorders first and **Excludes1** lets you know that borderline intellectual function, IQ above 70 to 84, should be coded R41.83 - not with one of these F codes.

Block F80-F89 is for pervasive and specific developmental disorders, such as problems with speech, language and math development disorders. **Block F90-F98** covers behavioral and emotional disorders with onset usually occurring in childhood and adolescence, but the condition sometimes continues throughout the patient's lifetime and may be treated in an adult. The code F99 *Mental disorder, not otherwise specified*, is used only when no other code is appropriate.

Are you psyched for some exercises? Let's get started!

5.1

Which of the following codes can be used to describe bipolar disorder?

_____ F45.8   _____ F31.11

_____ F03.91   _____ F51.3

5.2

Dr. Watson has an 86 year-old patient who has dementia, which involves diminished reasoning and thinking. Which code is for this condition?

_____ F45.8   _____ F31.11

_____ F03.91   _____ F51.3

5.3

A patient has physical symptoms, but all the medical tests are negative and Dr. Watson has not yet found a medical condition. Which code applies?

_____ F45.8   _____ F31.11

_____ F03.91   _____ F51.3

5.1

The answer is <u>F31.11</u>. Bipolar disorder is a mood [affective] disorder in which a person has periods of very high moods (formerly known as manic) and periods of low moods (also known as depressive). Look under the mood [affective] disorders block (**F30-F39**) for some more bipolar codes.

Bi- is Latin for double and *-polar* is Latin for opposite (in character or in action).

5.2

<u>F03.91</u> *Unspecified dementia, unspecified severity, with behavioral disturbance* is the correct code.

With dementia, reasoning is also affected, as is the person's ability to function in a normal daily life. One commonly known cause of dementia is Alzheimer's disease.

5.3

<u>F45.8</u> is the code that refers to a somatoform disorder, a mental disorder in which no physical condition or injury can be found that explains the patient's symptoms. *Soma-* is from the Greek word for the body; *-form* is from Latin for having the form of.

QUICK QUIZ Answers in Appendix A

_____ 5.1 Used as a placeholder	*A.* The letter X
_____ 5.2 Gives examples of content	*B.* **Excludes2** note
_____ 5.3 Cannot be coded at the same time	*C.* **Excludes1** note
_____ 5.4 Both conditions can be coded	*D.* **Includes** note

_____ 5.5 Endocrine Diseases	*A.* Codes begin with L
_____ 5.6 Circulatory System	*B.* Codes begin with I
_____ 5.7 Factors Influencing Health Status	*C.* Codes begin with E
_____ 5.8 Skin and Subcutaneous	*D.* Codes begin with Z

5.4

Which code below covers anxiety, a condition of uneasiness, worry and even dread? Maybe you've experienced it while preparing for a test.

_____ F30.3   _____ F23

_____ F41.1   _____ F44.81

5.5

Which of these codes is used for psychosis?

_____ F30.3   _____ F23

_____ F41.1   _____ F44.81

5.6

Which code is for dissociative disorder, a condition that involves a disruption of memory, perception or awareness?

_____ F30.3   _____ F23

_____ F41.1   _____ F44.81

5.7

Which of these terms, used in **Block F30-F39**, refers to moods and feelings?

_____ Affective   _____ Psychosis

_____ Anxiety   _____ Dissociative disorder

5.8

Which large block in the ICD-10 covers mental and behavioral disorders due to psychoactive substance use?

_____ **Block F01-F09**

_____ **Block F10-F19**

_____ **Block F20-F29**

5.4

The correct answer is <u>F41.1</u>.

Code F40 covers anxiety about things like spiders, thunderstorms, bridges and blood. F41 covers panic attacks and other anxieties.

5.5

The correct answer is <u>F23</u>.

Psych- means mind. *-osis* means condition or sickness. Psychosis is a generic term for a mental state with loss of contact with reality. It literally means a sickness or unhealthy condition of the mind.

5.6

<u>F44.81</u> is a code for dissociative disorder.

Dissociative disorders are thought to be primarily caused by psychological trauma. Code F44.81 *Dissociative identity disorder*, formerly called multiple personality disorder, may be diagnosed when the individual exhibits two or more distinct personalities.

5.7

<u>Affective</u> is the correct answer.

This block is for mood [affective] disorders. Notice that several kinds of disorders are listed here, including manic, bipolar, depressive, and mood disorders.

5.8

The correct answer is **Block F10-F19**.

Scan through this block and note that it is important to specify the substance. Various substances listed include: alcohol, opioids, cannabis, sedatives, cocaine, other stimulants, hallucinogens, nicotine, inhalants, and other psychoactive substances.

5.9

Which of the following disorders are included in this chapter?

_____ Schizophrenia   _____ Mood disorders

_____ Anxiety   _____ Stress-related disorders

_____ Adult personality disorders   _____ Developmental disorders

_____ All of these

5.10

Codes for nonpsychotic mental disorders begin with which letter?

_____ E   _____ F   _____ G   _____ H

5.11

Should the diagnosis of a mental disorder with hallucinations that is due to an exogenous toxic substance be reported using an F06 code?

_____ Yes   _____ No

5.12

Endocrine, nutritional and metabolic diseases codes begin with which letter(s)?

_____ A   _____ B   _____ C   _____ D   _____ E   _____ F

5.13

Neoplasms codes begin with which letter(s)?

_____ A   _____ B   _____ C   _____ D   _____ E   _____ F

5.14

Diseases of the blood and blood-forming organs codes begin with which letter(s)?

_____ A   _____ B   _____ C   _____ D   _____ E   _____ F

5.9

The correct answer is <u>all of these</u>. All mental, behavioral, and neurodevelopmental disorders are included in this chapter.

5.10

Codes for nonpsychotic mental disorders (and all mental, behavioral, and neurodevelopmental disorders) begin with the letter <u>F</u>.

5.11

<u>Yes</u>, mental disorders with hallucinations due to an exogenous toxic substance should be reported using an F06 code.

You know that because the **Includes** note after F06 specifically covers mental disorders due to exogenous toxic substance.

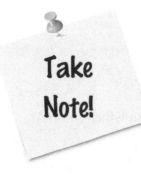

An **Includes** note is a coder's friend!
It further defines or gives examples of
the content of the category.

5.12

Codes for endocrine, nutritional and metabolic diseases begin with the letter <u>E</u>.

5.13

Codes for neoplasms begin with <u>either C or D.</u>

5.14

Codes for diseases of the blood and blood-forming organs begin with the letter <u>D</u>.

5.15

Certain infectious and parasitic diseases codes begin with which letter(s)?

_____ A   _____ B   _____ C   _____ D   _____ E   _____ F

5.16

Look at the first indented categories after codes F10 through F16 and also F18 and F19. What order do the categories follow?

_____ Abuse, unspecified, dependence
_____ Dependence, abuse unspecified
_____ Abuse, dependence, unspecified
_____ Unspecified, dependence, abuse

5.17

Look at the block covering schizophrenia, schizotypal, delusional, and other non-mood psychotic disorders. Which two categories are further broken down?

_____ F20 and F21   _____ F20 and F22   _____ F20 and F23
_____ F20 and F24   _____ F20 and F25   _____ F20 and F28

5.18

Take a look at the block for intellectual disabilities. How are these categories organized?

_____ Age of patient   _____ Severity of disability

5.19

The doctor noted code F94.0 on a bill for a 37 year-old man. Is this an appropriate code since he is an adult?

_____ Yes   _____ No

5.15

Codes for certain infectious and parasitic diseases begin with <u>either A or B</u>.

5.16

The categories follow this order: <u>abuse, dependence, unspecified</u>.

All of these codes are for substance abuse. The block is labeled **F10-F19** (Mental and behavioral disorders due to psychoactive substance use). Did you notice that our question skipped F17 *Nicotine dependence*? Why? Because the codes beginning with F17 are categorized differently. They are by type of tobacco product.

5.17

The two categories that are further broken down are <u>F20 and F25</u>.

F20 *Schizophrenia* is broken down by type: paranoid, disorganized, catatonic, undifferentiated and residual. F25 *Schizoaffective disorders* is also broken down by type: bipolar type and depressive type. Both codes also have the catch-all categories "other" and "unspecified."

5.18

The categories in the block for intellectual disabilities are organized by <u>severity of disability</u>.

The categories are ordered mild, moderate, severe and then profound followed by the last two "other" and "unspecified." Notice that these are ranked primarily by IQ levels.

5.19

<u>Yes</u>, code F94.0 can be used with an adult.

Code F94.0 is in **Block F90-F98** (Behavioral and emotional disorders with onset usually occurring in childhood and adolescence). But below the block title a note says the codes within this block can be used regardless of the patient's age.

Chapter Quiz (Answers in Appendix A)

Match the terms to their definitions. Some of the Greek and Latin terms from this chapter are bold. Hint: see the handy list in Appendix B.

_____ 5.1	Periods of high and low moods	A. **Psych**osis
_____ 5.2	Uneasiness and worry	B. Dementia
_____ 5.3	Disruption of memory or perception	C. Affective
_____ 5.4	Symptoms but no medical condition	D. **Psych**oactive
_____ 5.5	A drug that affects the mental state	E. Anxiety
_____ 5.6	Diminished capacity to think	F. **Soma**toform
_____ 5.7	Refers to feelings and emotions	G. Dissociative disorder
_____ 5.8	Unhealthy condition of the mind	H. Bi**polar**

Find the code for each diagnosis.

_____ 5.9	Agoraphobia with panic disorder	A. F32.1
_____ 5.10	Major depressive disorder	B. F20.0
_____ 5.11	Amnestic disorder	C. F60.2
_____ 5.12	Anorexia nervosa, unspecified	D. F31.63
_____ 5.13	Alcohol abuse	E. F94.0
_____ 5.14	Manic episode in full remission	F. F04
_____ 5.15	Selective mutism	G. F41.9
_____ 5.16	Anxiety disorder, unspecified	H. F10.151
_____ 5.17	Paranoid schizophrenia	I. F44.2
_____ 5.18	Antisocial personality disorder	J. F40.01
_____ 5.19	Bipolar disorder, current episode	K. F50.00
_____ 5.20	Dissociative stupor	L. F30.4

Match the code to the block title the code is in.

_____ 5.21 F31.75	A. Mental disorders due to known physiological conditions
_____ 5.22 F72	B. Mental and behavioral disorders due to psychoactive substance use
_____ 5.23 F51.3	C. Schizophrenia, schizotypal, delusional, and other non-mood psychotic disorders
_____ 5.24 F99	D. Mood [affective] disorders
_____ 5.25 F06.2	E. Anxiety, dissociative, stress-related, somatoform and other nonpsychotic mental disorders
_____ 5.26 F63.2	F. Behavioral syndromes associated with physiological disturbances and physical factors
_____ 5.27 F25.1	G. Disorders of adult personality and behavior
_____ 5.28 F41.1	H. Intellectual disabilities
_____ 5.29 F80.1	I. Pervasive and specific development disorders
_____ 5.30 F16.251	J. Behavioral and emotional disorders with onset usually occurring in childhood and adolescence
_____ 5.31 F90.1	K. Unspecified mental disorder

Indicate all appropriate notes for each code. All of these codes have more than one note and notes may be used more than once. Be sure to check the notes at the beginning of the chapter, as well as before the blocks and categories.

5.32 F42.2 _____ _____	A. **Includes** note
5.33 F14.120 _____ _____ _____	B. **Excludes1** note
5.34 F64.1 _____ _____ _____ _____	C. **Excludes2** note
5.35 F23 _____ _____	D. **"Use additional code"** note
5.36 F02.81 _____ _____ _____ _____	E. **"Code first"** note
5.37 F84.2 _____ _____ _____	
5.38 F32.3 _____ _____ _____	

6

Diseases of the Nervous System

The nervous system consists of two main parts: the central nervous system, which is the brain and spinal cord, and the peripheral nervous system, the nerves that run throughout the body.

The peripheral nervous system is divided into two parts: the autonomic nervous system which acts mostly below the level of awareness, such as breathing or digestion, and the somatic system, which controls the voluntary muscles.

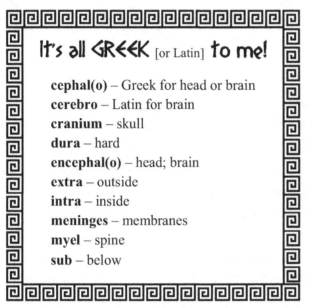

It's all GREEK [or Latin] to me!

cephal(o) – Greek for head or brain
cerebro – Latin for brain
cranium – skull
dura – hard
encephal(o) – head; brain
extra – outside
intra – inside
meninges – membranes
myel – spine
sub – below

The first block in this chapter is G00-G09 (Inflammatory diseases of the central nervous system). The membranes that cover and protect the brain and spinal cord are called meninges. So, even if you've never seen the word, you may guess that when the meninges become inflamed it is called meningitis. As you remember, *-itis* means inflammation.

Find G04 *Encephalitis, myelitis and encephalomyelitis* in your book. *Myel-* is from the Greek for spine. Myelitis is inflammation of the spine.

Here is a long word, but you know all the parts: encephalomyelitis. The Greek word for brain is *encephalo-*, so encephalitis is inflammation of the brain and encephalomyelitis means inflammation of the brain and spinal cord.

The medical term for the skull is the Latin word *cranium*. The prefix *intra-* means inside and the prefix *extra-* means outside. Both come from Latin. Put *intra-* and *cranium* together and you get intracranial, which means inside the skull.

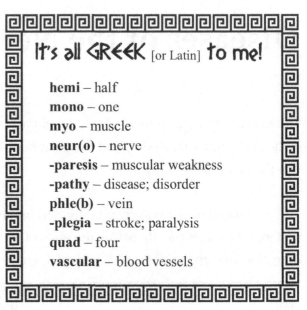

It's all GREEK [or Latin] **to me!**

hemi – half
mono – one
myo – muscle
neur(o) – nerve
-paresis – muscular weakness
-pathy – disease; disorder
phle(b) – vein
-plegia – stroke; paralysis
quad – four
vascular – blood vessels

In the Greek and Latin box here, you'll see some more root words that appear often in this chapter.

Cerebro- is another word part that means brain, but it comes from a Latin word. Cerebrospinal refers to the brain and the spinal cord while cerebrovascular refers to the brain and blood vessels. *Vascular* refers to blood vessels.

Although chapter 9 of the ICD-10 book includes the vascular system, some diagnoses in this chapter relate to veins. G08, for example is *Intracranial and intraspinal phlebitis and thrombophlebitis*. *Thrombo-* means a clot. The term *phleb-* is from a Greek word meaning vein, so you can deduce that phlebitis is inflammation of a vein and thrombophlebitis is inflammation of a vein caused by a clot. This is where a basic knowledge of root words comes in handy and makes coding fun!

For example, in **Block G50-G59** (Nerve, nerve root and plexus disorders) you will find the mononeuropathy codes (G56-G59). *Mono-* is a prefix from Greek meaning one. *Neuro-* is from Greek and means nerve. The suffix *-pathy* also comes from Greek and means disease or disorder. Mononeuropathy is a disease involving one nerve. The next block includes the polyneuropathy codes (**G60-G65**). *Poly-* is a prefix from Greek for many. Polyneuropathy, is a disease involving more than one nerve.

In the next block, **G70-G73** (Diseases of myoneural junction and muscle), you will find code G72 *Other and unspecified myopathies*. *Myo-* comes from the Greek word for muscle, so, myopathy is a disease of the muscles.

Locate codes G81 *Hemiplegia and hemiparesis* and G82 *Paraplegia (paraparesis) and quadriplegia (quadriparesis)* in **Block G80-G83** (Cerebral palsy and other paralytic syndromes). *Hemi-* means half and *-paresis* means muscular weakness. So, hemiparesis is muscular weakness on one side of the body and *quad-* means four, so quadriparesis is muscular weakness in all four limbs. The similar term *-plegia* comes from a Greek word meaning stroke or paralysis. Hemiplegia is paralysis of one side, or half of the body. Quadriplegia is paralysis of all four limbs.

Deciphering root words, prefixes and suffixes is like a game, isn't it! Let's practice what you just learned. Feel free to refer to the Greek and Latin boxes.

6.1
Which term in the first two blocks refers to the brain and spinal cord?

_____ Central nervous system   _____ Autonomic nervous system
_____ Peripheral nervous system

6.2
According to the codes in **Block G60-G65**, which term refers to the part of the nervous system consisting of the nerves leading to the spinal cord and brain?

_____ Central nervous system   _____ Autonomic nervous system
_____ Peripheral nervous system

6.3
Based on your knowledge of basic root words so far, what do the terms *extra-* and *intra-* mean?

_____ Outside and inside   _____ Hard and soft
_____ Left and right

6.4
Which of these codes applies to mononeuropathy, a disease of one nerve?

_____ G56.01   _____ G62.81
_____ G72.0   _____ G04.30

6.1

The <u>central nervous system</u> (CNS) consists of the brain and spinal cord.

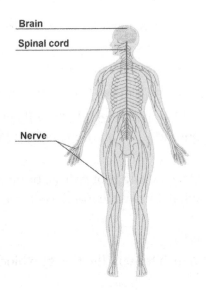

6.2

The <u>peripheral nervous system</u> refers to the outlying nerves that lead to the central nervous system.

6.3

The correct answer is <u>outside and inside</u>.

Extra- means outside and *intra-* means inside.

6.4

The answer is <u>G56.01</u>.

You can answer this because you learned that *mono-* means one, *neuro-* means nerve, and *-pathy* is a disease or disorder. Codes G56 and G57 are examples of mononeuropathy conditions.

QUICK QUIZ Answers in Appendix A

_____ 6.1	External causes of morbidity	*A.* Codes begin with T
_____ 6.2	Injury, poisoning and certain other consequences of external causes	*B.* Codes begin with V
_____ 6.3	Diseases of the musculoskeletal system and connective tissue	*C.* Codes begin with M
_____ 6.4	Congenital malformations, deformation and chromosomal abnormalities	*D.* Codes begin with Q

6.5

Which of these codes should be used for a diagnosis of polyneuropathy, which indicates that more than one nerve is affected?

_____ G56.01   _____ G62.81
_____ G72.0   _____ G04.30

6.6

Myopathy means a disease of the muscles. Which of these codes falls under the category for "Other and unspecified myopathies"?

_____ G56.01   _____ G62.81
_____ G72.0   _____ G04.30

6.7

Which of these codes describes a disease of the brain called encephalopathy?

_____ G56.01   _____ G62.81
_____ G72.0   _____ G04.30

6.8

A newborn has hydrocephalus, a condition in which there is an abnormal amount of cerebrospinal fluid in the brain. Which code should you use for hydrocephalus?

_____ G40.201   _____ G91.1
_____ G81.12   _____ G82.53

There's a code for THAT??

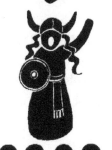

What danger could possibly lurk in the opera house? Only The Phantom knows! But ICD-10 is prepared! Check out code Y92.253.

6.5

G62.81 is a polyneuropathy code.

Poly- means many. *neuro-* means nerve and *-pathy* is a disease or disorder. **Block G60-G65** is for polyneuropathies.

6.6

G72.0 is for drug-induced myopathy.

Myo- means muscle. As you know, *-pathy* means disease or disorder. There are many causes of and body parts affected by myopathy, such as in Chapter 9, which includes myopathy of the heart.

6.7

G04.30 is one of the encephalopathy codes.

Encephal(o)- refers to the brain. *-pathy* means disease or disorder. Using the alphabetical index of your ICD-10, look up encephalopathy. You will find many different kinds of encephalopathy and they are located in different chapters throughout the book. Many are G codes located in this chapter.

Take Note! Sometimes when combining Greek and Latin roots to make a medical term, inserting a vowel between them makes the word easier to pronounce. The most common additional vowel is "o," but other vowels are also used. Notice encephalopathy above. The Greek word part is **encephal**. But to make it easier to say, an "o" is added and you have encephalopathy.

6.8

G91.1 is for obstructive hydrocephalus.

Hydro- means water (cerebrospinal fluid). *-cephalus* refers to the brain. Hydrocephalus is most common in infants.

6.9

Mr. Jones had an epileptic seizure while at his doctor's office. Which category applies?

_____ G40   _____ G81
_____ G82   _____ G91

6.10

Sally's doctor's notes indicate that she has spastic hemiplegia (paralysis) affecting the entire left dominant side of her body. Which code applies?

_____ G81.91   _____ G81.13
_____ G81.12   _____ G81.92

6.11

Josef was involved in a car crash and now has quadriplegia. Which of these categories will you use?

_____ G40   _____ G81
_____ G82   _____ G91

6.12

One of Dr. Able's patients has developed encephalitis, a viral inflammation of the brain. Into which of these categories does encephalitis fall?

_____ G00   _____ G04
_____ G11   _____ G07

6.13

The patient's inflammation has spread. It is now an inflammation of the brain and spinal cord. The doctor's diagnosis is now "postinfectious acute disseminated encephalitis and encephalomyelitis." Which code should you use?

_____ G04.01   _____ G04.31
_____ G04.81   _____ G04.91

6.9

G40.201 is for epilepsy, which is characterized by seizures.

Seizures can be associated with a number of causes so not all seizures are covered in Diseases of the Nervous System. Look at G40 in your ICD-10 and notice the indented codes. ICD-10 requires very specific codes when diagnosing epilepsy.

6.10

G81.12 *Spastic hemiplegia affecting left dominant side* is the correct answer.

Hemi- means half, *-plegia* means paralysis. It can be either the left side or the right side and ICD-10 instructs you to code the affected side.

6.11

G82 covers quadriplegia.

Quad- means four and *-plegia* means paralysis. Quadriplegia is paralysis of all four limbs.

6.12

G04 is the category for encephalitis, myelitis and encephalomyelitis.

You already know these word parts. A smart coder breaks medical terms into their parts to help know what they mean and speed up the coding process. *Encephal-* means the brain, *myel-* is the spine and *-itis* means inflammation. Look at G04 and G05 in the ICD-10.

6.13

G04.01 *Postinfectious acute disseminated encephalitis and encephalomyelitis* is the best answer.

Look at the word parts. *Encephal-* is the brain. *Myel-* is the spine. *-itis* means inflammation. Encephalomyelitis is described with codes G04 and G05.

6.14

Another patient has an inflammation of the spinal cord which the doctor has diagnosed as myelitis. What is the code for this condition?

_____ G03.1   _____ G08

_____ G04.91   _____ G04.9

6.15

Dr. Able's patient has pneumococcal meningitis, an acute inflammation of the membranes that cover and protect the brain and spinal cord. Which of these codes is best for this?

_____ G00.1   _____ G00.2

_____ G00.3   _____ G03.1

6.16

Check the Greek and Latin boxes for this chapter and decide which of these words means inside the cranium, or skull.

_____ Intracranial   _____ Phlebitis

_____ Thrombophlebitis   _____ Cerebrovascular

6.17

Some diseases affect the blood vessels of the brain. Based on the word parts what term do you think refers to the blood vessels of the brain?

_____ Intracranial   _____ Phlebitis

_____ Thrombophlebitis   _____ Cerebrovascular

6.18

Mr. Onassis has been diagnosed with phlebitis. Using the Greek and Latin boxes, what is the best definition of phlebitis?

_____ many veins involved   _____ inflammation of a vein

_____ a flea bite   _____ the study of veins

6.14

<u>G04.91</u> is a myelitis code.

Myel- means the spinal cord and *-itis* means inflammation.

6.15

<u>G00.1</u> is for pneumococcal meningitis.

The meninges are listed under codes G00, G01, G02 and G03. Meningitis is classified by cause and the choices are bacterial, infectious and parasitic, and due to other causes.

6.16

<u>Intracranial</u> means inside the cranium, or skull.

Intra- means inside and *cranial* refers to the cranium or skull. For example, if the doctor's diagnosis is intracranial abscess and granuloma, the code is G06.0.

6.17

<u>Cerebrovascular</u> refers to the blood vessels in the brain.

The word parts: *cerebro-* means the brain. *-vascular* refers to the blood vessels. For example, code G46 *Vascular syndromes of brain in cerebrovascular diseases.*

6.18

<u>Phlebitis</u> means an inflammation of a vein.

Phleb- means vein and you know that *-itis* means inflammation.

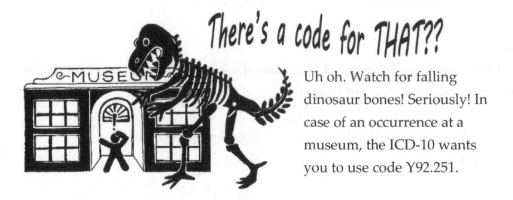

There's a code for THAT??

Uh oh. Watch for falling dinosaur bones! Seriously! In case of an occurrence at a museum, the ICD-10 wants you to use code Y92.251.

6.19

Ms. Blumenthal has been diagnosed with inflammation in a vein because of a blood clot. Use your Greek and Latin knowledge and decide which word applies.

_____ Intracranial   _____ Phlebitis

_____ Thrombophlebitis   _____ Cerebrovascular

6.20

Which letter applies to codes for diseases of the nervous system?

_____ F   _____ G   _____ H   _____ I

6.21

Are codes for encephalitis found in the nervous system section?

_____ Yes   _____ No

6.22

Are codes for cerebral palsy found in the nervous system section?

_____ Yes   _____ No

6.23

Are codes for meningitis found in the nervous system section?

_____ Yes   _____ No

6.24

Are codes for Parkinson's disease included in the nervous system?

_____ Yes   _____ No

6.19

Thromb(o)- means blood clot. Add it to phlebitis and you have <u>thrombophlebitis</u> – inflammation in a vein because of a blood clot.

Many times both phlebitis and thrombophlebitis are listed on the same code. Look at code G08. It is for *Intracranial and intraspinal phlebitis and thrombophlebitis.*

6.20

Codes for diseases of the nervous system begin with <u>G</u>.

They range from G00 to G99.

6.21

<u>Yes</u>, codes for encephalitis are found in the nervous system section.

Codes for encephalitis begin with G04 and G05. Encephalitis is an infection of the brain and the brain is part of the nervous system.

6.22

<u>Yes</u>, codes for cerebral palsy are found in the nervous system section.

Codes for cerebral palsy begin with G80. Cerebral palsy is a disorder caused by damage to the brain, and the brain is part of the nervous system.

6.23

<u>Yes</u>, codes for meningitis are found in the nervous system section.

Meningitis codes are G00-G03. Meningitis is a disease caused by the inflammation of the protective membranes covering the brain and spinal cord.

6.24

<u>Yes</u>, codes for Parkinson's disease are included in the nervous system.

Codes for Parkinson's disease begin with G20 and G21. Parkinson's disease is a disease of the brain.

6.25

What are the first three letters of codes for epilepsy?

_____ G39   _____ G40   _____ G41   _____ G42

6.26

The patient has acute pyelonephritis. The cause of this patient's condition is a staphylococcus infection. Which is the proper way to list the codes?

_____ N10 followed by B95.61   _____ B95.61 followed by N10

6.27

The neurologist sees a new patient who was referred by her primary care physician. The patient has chronic meningitis. What is the code for this diagnosis?

_____

6.28

The patient has late onset Alzheimer's disease with dementia and behavioral disturbance. The experienced coder in the office shows two diagnosis codes, G30.1 and F02.811, on the bill. Is it ok to include both of these codes on one bill?

_____ Yes   _____ No

6.29

A newborn infant has congenital central alveolar hypoventilation syndrome, a type of sleep apnea. The new coder is trying to decide if G47.35 is the correct code. Read the notes and give your answer.

_____ Yes   _____ No

6.25

Codes for epilepsy begin with <u>G40</u>.

Look through these codes and notice the difference in localization, generalized, absence and juvenile. This is the main way these codes are divided.

6.26

The codes should be listed as <u>N10 followed by B95.61</u>.

Look up N10, the code for acute pyelonephritis. There is a **"Use additional code"** note specifically mentioning B95 – B97 as an additional code.

6.27

The code for chronic meningitis is <u>G03.1</u>.

Did you look up meningitis and then under it look for chronic in the alphabetical index. Next, you must go to the tabular list (chapter) to look for notes.

6.28

<u>Yes</u>, it is ok to include both G30.1 and F02.81- on the same bill.

Read the note under the category G30 *Alzheimer's disease*. It specifically says to use an additional code to identify dementia with behavioral disturbance. This includes F02.811.

6.29

<u>No</u>, congenital central alveolar hypoventilation syndrome should not be coded as G47.35.

Why not? Read the notes after G47.3 *Sleep Apnea*. There is an **Excludes1** note that says sleep apnea of newborns should be coded P28.3. The P codes are for certain conditions originating during the perinatal period. G47.3 is for use with all patients except newborns.

Chapter Quiz (Answers in Appendix A)

Using your new knowledge of Greek and Latin roots, match the definitions to the terms. Some of the Greek and Latin terms from this chapter are bold.

_____ 6.1	Generic term for disease of the muscles	A. Hydro**cephal**us
_____ 6.2	Weakness in half of the body	B. Neuro**pathy**
_____ 6.3	Inside the cranium or skull	C. Mono**neuro**pathy
_____ 6.4	Inflammation of the brain	D. **Mening**itis
_____ 6.5	Inflammation of a vein	E. Encephalo**myel**itis
_____ 6.6	Blood clot in a vein	F. Cerebro**vascular**
_____ 6.7	Malfunction of a single nerve	G. **Intra**cranial
_____ 6.8	An abnormal amount of cerebrospinal fluid in the brain	H. Hemi**paresis**
		I. Thrombo**phleb**itis
_____ 6.9	Inflammation of the brain and spinal cord	J. **Myel**itis
_____ 6.10	Disease of a nerve	K. Encephalo**pathy**
_____ 6.11	Paralysis of half of the body	L. **Encephal**itis
_____ 6.12	Inflammation of the spinal cord	M. Myo**pathy**
_____ 6.13	Refers to blood vessels of the brain	N. **Phleb**itis
_____ 6.14	Inflammation of the membranes that protect the brain and spinal cord	O. Poly**neuro**pathy
		P. Hemi**plegia**
_____ 6.15	Disease of the brain	
_____ 6.16	More than one nerve is affected	

Use the alphabetical index to find the code for each description.

_____ 6.17   Drug induced tic

_____ 6.18   Epileptic spasms, not intractable, without status epilepticus

_____ 6.19   Subacute necrotizing myelitis of central nervous system

_____ 6.22   Obstructive hydrocephalus

_____ 6.21   Postimmunization acute disseminated encephalitis, myelitis and encephalomyelitis

_____ 6.22   Radiation-induced polyneuropathy

_____ 6.23   Flaccid hemiplegia affecting right dominant side

_____ 6.24   Hereditary spastic paraplegia

_____ 6.25   Muscular dystrophy

_____ 6.26   Lesion of sciatic nerve, right lower limb

_____ 6.27   Degeneration of nervous system due to alcohol

Fill in the blank with the first letter(s) of the codes that go with each chapter.

_____ 6.28 Certain conditions originating in the perinatal period	A or B
_____ 6.29 Factors influencing health status	C or D
_____ 6.30 Neoplasms	E
_____ 6.31 Diseases of the ear and mastoid process	F
_____ 6.32 Genitourinary system	H
_____ 6.33 Certain infectious and parasitic diseases	L
_____ 6.34 Endocrine, nutritional and metabolic	N
_____ 6.35 Mental, behavioral and neurodevelopmental	P
_____ 6.36 Skin and subcutaneous tissue	Z

7

Diseases of the Eye and Adnexa

Chapter 7 deals with diseases and conditions of the eye. Let's take a look.

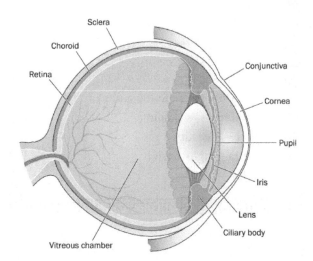

This chapter is organized first by parts of the eye, followed by diseases and conditions related to the eye. Note the word *adnexa*. It comes from the Latin meaning accessory. So the eyelid and the optic nerve, for example, are considered accessories of the eye. Let's examine the blocks and take note of some terminology relating to diseases of the eye and adnexa.

The first block is **H00-H05** (Disorders of the eyelid, lacrimal system and orbit). Example diagnoses are H02.4 *Ptosis of eyelid* (*ptosis* comes from Greek and means to drop downward) and H01.0 *Blepharitis*. **Blephar-** comes from the Greek word for eyelid. H04 is *Disorders of lacrimal system*. The lacrimal system creates tears. H05 is *Disorders of orbit*. The orbit is the bony part of the skull that contains the eyeball.

H10-H11 (Disorders of conjunctiva) is the second block. The conjunctiva (from the Latin word meaning "join together") is the mucous membrane that lines the eyelid and reflects onto the eyeball. Find code H10 *Conjunctivitis*: **conjunctiv-** and *-itis* (inflammation).

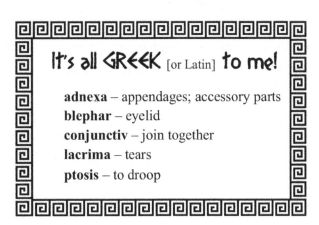

It's all GREEK [or Latin] to me!

adnexa – appendages; accessory parts
blephar – eyelid
conjunctiv – join together
lacrima – tears
ptosis – to droop

Block H15-H22 covers disorders of sclera, cornea, iris and ciliary body. The word sclera comes from Greek and means hard. The sclera is a tough fibrous tissue that covers the white of the eye. Now, find code H18.44 *Keratomalacia*. **Kerato-** is from Greek and refers to the cornea, **-malacia** means softening. So, keratomalacia is softening of the cornea. Cornea comes from the Latin word *cornu*, which means horn. It is the clear, transparent portion of the eye that helps focus images and light onto the retina.

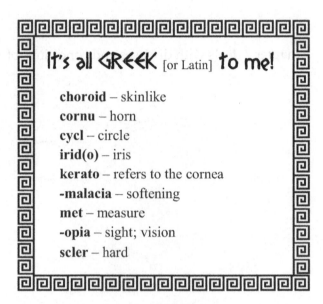

It's all GREEK [or Latin] to me!

choroid – skinlike
cornu – horn
cycl – circle
irid(o) – iris
kerato – refers to the cornea
-malacia – softening
met – measure
-opia – sight; vision
scler – hard

Note on the Greek chart that *irido-* means the iris and *cycl-* means circle. Therefore, code H20 *Iridocyclitis* is inflammation of the iris and ciliary body, a ring-shaped tissue inside the eye. The ciliary body is located behind the iris.

The lens, along with the cornea, focuses the light rays so they form a perfect image on the retina, similar to focusing a camera. You'll find codes for disorders of lens in **Block H25-H28**. Most codes in this block are for cataracts.

Block H30-H36 is for disorders of choroid and retina. The choroid is a vascular coat around the eye and the retina receives images formed by the lens. Look up code H30 *Chorioretinal inflammation*. When you combine the terms choroid and retina you get chorioretinal.

You'll find glaucoma, a group of eye diseases which lead to damage of the optic nerve and vision loss, in **Block H40-H42**.

The vitreous body is a transparent jelly-like substance that fills the cavity of the eyeball. The eyeball is also referred to as the globe. Locate **Block H43-H44** (Disorders of vitreous body and globe). You'll remember that hemorrhage means a leakage of blood. Find H43.1 *Vitreous hemorrhage* in your ICD-10 code book. This is a condition in which blood leaks into the vitreous body.

Look at code H46 *Optic neuritis*. Neuritis is made up of **neur-** which means nerve and **-itis** which means inflammation. Optic neuritis is inflammation of the optic nerve. **Block H46-H47** covers disorders of optic nerve and visual pathways.

The next two blocks, **H49-H52** and **H53-H54**, cover codes related to vision. **H49-H52** covers disorders of ocular muscles, binocular movement, accommodation and refraction. **H53-H54** covers visual disturbances and blindness.

Knowing the parts of medical terms helps you understand them. For example, see H52.0 *Hypermetropia*. It's a long word but it is made of three Greek word parts: **hyper-** meaning extra, **met-** referring to measurement and **-opia** referring to vision. So hypermetropia means extra distance vision which is farsightedness.

After you answer these questions about the eye, you'll see everything more clearly!

7.1

Les has anterior scleritis of the left eye. Which code best fits this condition?

_____ H05.002   _____ H05.011   _____ H15.012

7.2

Which of these codes would you use for a retinal detachment with single break, left eye?

_____ H33.011   _____ H33.012   _____ H33.022

7.3

Which of these codes would you use for atrophy of bilateral orbit?

_____ H05.311   _____ H05.312   _____ H05.313

7.4

Which code is for degeneration of the iris in the right eye?

_____ H21.231   _____ H21.232   _____ H21.233

7.1

H15.012 is the best code for anterior scleritis of the left eye.

H15.002 is not a good choice because it is for "unspecified" and this patient has anterior. H15.011 is not a good choice because it is for the right eye and this patient's condition is for the left eye.

7.2

H33.012 is the correct answer because it specifies left eye.

H33.011 is wrong because it specifies right eye and H33.022 doesn't work because it covers multiple breaks and this patient has a single break.

7.3

H05.313 specifies bilateral (both eyes).

H05.311 doesn't work because it specifies right orbit and H05.312 is wrong because it specifies left orbit. The orbit is the bony cavity of the skull that contains the eyeball. *Disorders of orbit* are H05 in the ICD-10.

7.4

The code for degeneration of the iris (pigmentary), right eye is H21.231.

The other choices are wrong because H21.322 is for left eye and H21.233 is for bilateral (both eyes).

QUICK QUIZ *Answers in Appendix A*

_____ 7.1 Diseases of the Circulatory System	**A.**	Codes begin with S
_____ 7.2 Injury, Poisoning and Certain Other Consequences of External Causes	**B.**	Codes begin with I
_____ 7.3 External Causes of Morbidity	**C.**	Codes begin with L
_____ 7.4 Diseases of the Skin and Subcutaneous Tissue	**D.**	Codes begin with W

7.5

Which of these codes is for a corneal abscess of the right eye?

_____ H16.311   _____ H16.312   _____ H16.313   _____ H16.319

7.6

The patient has simple chronic conjunctivitis of both eyes. Which code is that?

_____ H10.421   _____ H10.422   _____ H10.423   _____ H10.429

7.7

The patient has dry eye syndrome of the left lacrimal gland. Select the best code.

_____ H04.121   _____ H04.122   _____ H04.123   _____ H04.129

7.8

Dr. Sharp's patient has an anterior dislocation of the lens of the right eye. Which code best describes this condition?

_____ H27.131   _____ H27.121
_____ H27.132   _____ H27.122

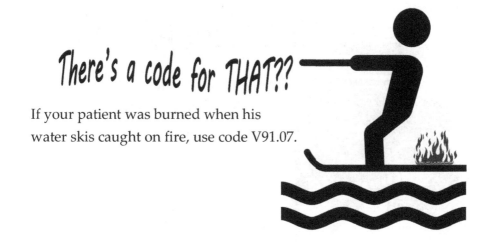

There's a code for THAT??

If your patient was burned when his water skis caught on fire, use code V91.07.

7.5

H16.311 is the code for corneal abscess of the right eye.

Codes H16, H17 and H18 are for conditions related to the cornea. The prefix *kerato-* refers to the cornea.

7.6

H10.423 is the code for chronic conjunctivitis of both eyes.

Disorders of conjunctiva are in **Block H10-H11.**

7.7

H04.122 is for dry eye syndrome of the left lacrimal gland.

Look at H04 and the indented codes beneath it. Believe it or not, there are more than 100 codes covering disorders of the lacrimal system.

7.8

H27.121 is the best code for anterior dislocation of the lens of the right eye.

You'll find the codes for disorders of the lens in **Block H25-H28.**

There's a code for THAT??

Housework has its ups and downs. Y93.E3 covers an activity involving vacuuming.

7.9

Jamie has age-related choroidal atrophy of both eyes. Which code best describes this condition?

_____ H31.111   _____ H31.113

_____ H31.112   _____ H31.119

7.10

Alexi has a hemorrhage of the vitreous body of the right eye. Select the best code for this condition.

_____ H43.00   _____ H43.11

_____ H43.10   _____ H43.12

7.11

Which code is for degeneration of the ciliary body of both eyes?

_____ H21.221   _____ H21.223

_____ H21.222   _____ H21.229

7.12

A patient has blepharitis, inflammation of their right lower eyelid. Which of these is the best code for this condition?

_____ H01.001   _____ H01.002   _____ H01.004

QUICK QUIZ Answers in Appendix A	
_____ 7.5 Over, bigger or enlarged	**A.** Hypo
_____ 7.6 Half	**B.** Sub
_____ 7.7 Under, smaller or reduced	**C.** Hyper
_____ 7.8 Below	**D.** Hemi

7.9

H31.113 is the code for age-related choroidal atrophy of both eyes.

Choroid is from a Greek word meaning skin-like. Look at **Block H30-H36**.

7.10

The best code for vitreous hemorrhage of the right eye is H43.11.

Vitreous is from the Latin for glassy. Look at **Block H43-H44**.

7.11

H21.223 is the code for degeneration of the ciliary body of both eyes.

The ciliary body codes are H20, H21 and H22.

7.12

H01.002 *Unspecified blepharitis right lower eyelid* is the best choice.

Blepharitis is inflammation of the eyelid. Blepharitis is made up of two major word parts: *Blephar-* which means eyelid and *-itis* which means inflammation.

QUICK QUIZ *Answers in Appendix A*

_____ 7.9 The codes should never be used at the same time	*A.*	Etiology/manifestation
_____ 7.10 Further defines (gives examples of) the content in a category	*B.*	**Excludes1** note
_____ 7.11 You must use a different code, but can be used at the same time	*C.*	**Excludes2** note
_____ 7.12 Tells you that the underlying condition should be coded first	*D.*	**Includes** note

7.13

A patient has ptosis, or drooping of his left eyelid. Which code is best for this condition?

_____ H02.401   _____ H02.402   _____ H02.403

7.14

Dr. Sharp is treating a young, malnourished child whose corneal tissue in the right eye is softening, a condition known as keratomalacia. Which code would you use?

_____ H18.441   _____ H18.442   _____ H18.443

7.15

Dr. Sharp sees a patient whose ciliary body and iris in both eyes are infected. He has diagnosed it as primary iridocyclitis. Which of these codes is appropriate?

_____ H20.011   _____ H20.012   _____ H20.013

7.16

Read through the Chapter-Specific Coding Guidelines in the ICD-10 that relate to Chapter 7. Which of the following block(s) have guidelines listed?

_____ Disorders of conjunctiva
_____ Disorders of lens
_____ Glaucoma
_____ Disorders of vitreous body and globe

7.17

Page through the chapter for diseases of the eye and adnexa. Look at the most detailed level of the diagnoses. What do most codes have in common?

_____ Other, non-specific
_____ Eye, adnexa
_____ Right eye, left eye, bilateral, unspecified eye

7.13

H02.402 is the code for unspecified ptosis of left eyelid.

Blepharoptosis is the condition in which one or both eyelids droop. *Blephar-* means eyelid. *Ptosis* means to drop, to move downward in position. Put them together and you have blepharoptosis.

7.14

H18.441 is for keratomalacia of the right eye.

Keratomalacia is the softening of the cornea. Keratomalacia is made of two parts: *kerato-* refers to the cornea, and *-malacia* means softening.

7.15

H20.013 is the code for primary iridocyclitis of both eyes.

Iridocyclitis means that the ciliary body and iris are infected. It is made of three major word parts: *irido-* means the iris, *cycl-* refers to the ciliary body, and *-itis* means infection or inflammation.

7.16

The Glaucoma block has information in the Chapter-Specific Coding Guidelines.

The guidelines for Diseases of the Eye and Adnexa are about glaucoma and blindness. Remember: before choosing a code, always check the Chapter-Specific Coding Guidelines.

7.17

The most detailed level for most codes in this chapter is right eye, left eye, bilateral, unspecified eye.

There are some exceptions – for example codes that begin H00 and H01 – but most codes are broken down at the most detailed level by right eye, left eye, bilateral (both sides of the body) and unspecified eye.

7.18

What is the last code in the Eye and Adnexa chapter?

_____

7.19

You see a claim that has two diagnosis codes: H01.005 and H10.502. Is it ok to code the claim this way?

_____ Yes   _____ No

7.20

You see a claim that has two diagnosis codes: H02.512 and G24.5. Is it ok to code the claim this way?

_____ Yes   _____ No

7.21

You see a claim with three diagnosis codes: H02.812, Z18.2 and S00.251. Which pair of codes should NOT be used together?

_____ H02.812 and Z18.2   _____ H02.812 and S00.251

7.22

Dr. Sharp has hired a new coder. She codes H04.323 with P39.1. Is it ok to code the claim this way?

_____ Yes   _____ No

7.23

Dr. Sharp has put two diagnoses in the chart. You code both H05.51 and H44.631. Is it correct to code these together?

_____ Yes   _____ No

7.18

The last code in the Eye and Adnexa chapter is <u>H59.89</u> *Other postprocedural complications and disorders of eye and adnexa, not elsewhere classified*.

7.19

<u>No</u>, you cannot use any of the H01.0 codes with any of the H10.5 codes.

Why not? There is an **Excludes1** note after H01.0 which lists H10.5-.

7.20

<u>Yes</u>, H02.512 and G24.5 can be coded together.

Why? The **Excludes2** note after H02.5 lists G24.5. **Excludes2** notes indicate that the condition excluded is not part of the condition represented by the code. So, the two codes can be used together.

7.21

<u>H02.812 and S00.251</u> should not be coded together.

Why not? There is an **Excludes1** note after H02.81 that excludes coding any H02.81 code with any S00.25 codes. There also is a "**Use additional code**" note specifying that you should use the Z18.- codes to identify the type of retained foreign body.

7.22

<u>No</u>, H04.323 and P39.1 should not be coded together.

Why not? The **Excludes1** note after H04.3 tells you specifically to exclude P39.1 with the H04.3 codes.

7.23

<u>Yes</u>, H05.51 and H44.631 can be coded together.

Why? Code H44.631 is mentioned in an **Excludes2** note under H05.5. This means that you can code these two together.

7.24

Dr. Sharp's new coder has used H05.51 with H02.811. Is it ok to code these together?

_____ Yes   _____ No

7.25

Dr. Sharp's new coder used H05.51 with S05.41. Is it ok to code these together?

_____ Yes   _____ No

7.26

Dr. Sharp has diagnosed the patient's injury as a retained foreign body in the eye. It is a wood fragment. Which code(s) would you choose?

_____ H05.51   _____ Z18.33   _____ Both H05.51 and Z18.33

7.27

Does H40.60 require the use of a 7th character?

_____ Yes   _____ No

7.28

Dr. Sharp has diagnosed a patient with moderate stage pigmentary glaucoma of the left eye. Which is the correct way to code this?

_____ H40.132   _____ H40.1322

There's a code for THAT??

Code Y92.14 covers prison as a place of occurrence (makes sense). But wait! Look at the indented code, Y92.146 *Swimming pool of prison as place of occurrence.* Pretty cushy prison!

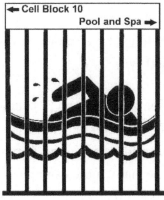

7.24

Yes, the new coder did his homework. H05.51 and H02.811 can be used together.

Why? Because code H02.81- is mentioned in an **Excludes2** note under H05.5, indicating that you can code these two together.

7.25

No, H05.51 and S05.41 cannot be coded together.

The new coder must have missed the **Excludes1** note under H05.5 which lists S05.4-. These codes cannot be listed together.

7.26

The answer is both H05.51 and Z18.33 should be coded together.

How do you know? The **"Use additional code"** note under H05.5 instructs you to identify the type of retained foreign body by using one of the Z18.- codes. Z18.33 is for retained wood fragments.

7.27

Yes, a 7th character is needed when using H40.60.

Why? Because there is a 7th character note following H40.6. Also, since H40.60 has only five characters, it requires one placeholder X. For example: H40.60X1 for mild stage. This is a perfect example of instructions regarding the 7th character. Take a few minutes now to review this fascinating subject of placeholders and 7th characters in the Basic Concepts Chapter.

7.28

H40.1322 is the correct way to code moderate stage pigmentary glaucoma of the left eye.

Some codes use a 7th character to further identify the diagnosis. For this code, the 7th character tells you the stage of the glaucoma. Moderate stage glaucoma is noted by adding a 2 in the 7th place of the code. Hence, H40.132 becomes H40.1322. You'll see many more examples of 7th characters in future exercises. Note: in this case, the code already had six characters, so a placeholder X is not necessary.

Chapter Quiz (Answers in Appendix A)

Match the definition to the word. Some of the Greek and Latin terms from this chapter are bold.

_____ 7.1	Softening of the cornea	A. Adnexa
_____ 7.2	Eyebrow or forehead drooping	B. Sclero**malacia**
_____ 7.3	Inflammation of the conjunctiva	C. **Blephar**itis
_____ 7.4	Accessories of the eye	D. **Conjunctiv**itis
_____ 7.5	Softening of the sclera	E. Brow **ptosis**
_____ 7.6	Inflammation of the eyelids	F. Kerato**malacia**

Enter Yes if the code requires the use of a 7th character.
Enter No if the code does NOT require the use of a 7th character.

_____ 7.7	H34.211		_____ 7.13	H40.10
_____ 7.8	H34.811		_____ 7.14	H40.112
_____ 7.9	H34.823		_____ 7.15	H40.152
_____ 7.10	H34.839		_____ 7.16	H40.213
_____ 7.11	H35.30		_____ 7.17	H40.60
_____ 7.12	H35.312		_____ 7.18	H40.822

Enter the number of placeholder Xs required for each code.
Enter 0 if none are required.
Enter No if the code doesn't require a 7th character.

_____ 7.19	H40.62		_____ 7.25	H40.219
_____ 7.20	H40.51		_____ 7.26	H40.20
_____ 7.21	H40.43		_____ 7.27	H40.10
_____ 7.22	H40.32		_____ 7.28	H35.329
_____ 7.23	H40.239		_____ 7.29	H34.833
_____ 7.24	H40.229		_____ 7.30	H34.811

Match the category to its description.

_____ 7.31	H26	A.	Retinal vascular occlusions
_____ 7.32	H53	B.	Intraoperative and postprocedural complications and disorders of eye and adnexa, NEC
_____ 7.33	H10	C.	Other cataract
_____ 7.34	H46	D.	Visual disturbances
_____ 7.35	H40	E.	Other inflammation of eyelid
_____ 7.36	H16	F.	Optic neuritis
_____ 7.37	H59	G.	Disorders of globe
_____ 7.38	H34	H.	Conjunctivitis
_____ 7.39	H44	I.	Nystagmus and other irregular eye movements
_____ 7.40	H52	J.	Glaucoma
_____ 7.41	H01	K.	Disorders of refraction and accommodation
_____ 7.42	H55	L.	Keratitis

Fill in the blank with the first letter(s) of the codes that go with each chapter.

_____ 7.43	Ear and Mastoid Process	A and B
_____ 7.44	Neoplasms	C and D
_____ 7.45	Mental and Behavioral	D
_____ 7.46	Nervous System	E
_____ 7.47	Blood and Immune Mechanisms	F
_____ 7.48	Certain Infectious & Parasitic Diseases	G
_____ 7.49	Digestive System	H
_____ 7.50	Endocrine, Nutritional and Metabolic	K

8

Diseases of the Ear and Mastoid Process

Listen up! We are about to explore coding for conditions and diseases of the external ear, the middle ear, and the inner ear.

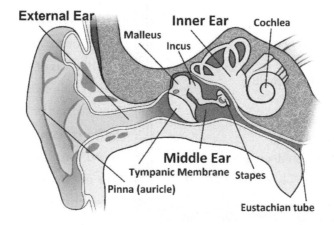

Before we start Chapter 8, let's get familiar with the notes at the beginning. A generic note tells you to first code the condition, and then use a second code to identify an external cause, if applicable. **Excludes2** lists some codes that may be used with codes in this chapter, but indicates that they should be listed separately.

The blocks at the beginning of Chapter 8 begin with **H60-H62** (Diseases of external ear). The first code in this chapter is H60 *Otitis externa*. *Ot-* comes from Greek and means the ear and *-itis* means inflammation, so otitis externa means inflammation of the external ear.

Now look at H61.1 *Noninfective disorders of pinna*. **Pinna** is from a Latin word meaning feather and refers to the external, or outer ear. It doesn't seem particularly logical that ear relates to feather, but both are appendages.

Moving down the codes, you will see H61.2 *Impacted cerumen*. **Cerumen** comes from the Latin word for wax. In this case it refers to ear wax.

Block H65-H75 (Diseases of middle ear and mastoid) begins with H65 *Nonsuppurative otitis media*. The term **suppurative** comes from a Latin word and means "forming pus." Nonsuppurative, then, means not producing pus. **Media** comes from the Latin word meaning medium or middle. Nonsuppurative otitis media is inflammation of the middle ear with no production of pus. The mastoid is a bone behind the ear, also called the mastoid process.

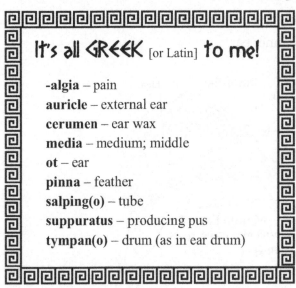

It's all GREEK [or Latin] to me!

-algia – pain
auricle – external ear
cerumen – ear wax
media – medium; middle
ot – ear
pinna – feather
salping(o) – tube
suppuratus – producing pus
tympan(o) – drum (as in ear drum)

Also part of the middle ear is the Eustachian tube. This tube extends from the middle ear to the pharynx and allows ventilation of the middle ear. Find H68 *Eustachian salpingitis and obstruction* in your book. *Salping-* comes from the Greek word for tube. Eustachian salpingitis is inflammation of the Eustachian tube.

Look at H72 *Perforation of tympanic membrane*. **Tympan-** is from a Greek word that means drum. So, the tympanic membrane is the eardrum. It separates the middle ear from the outer ear. Sometimes there are two medical terms for the same body part. For example, the term **myring-** is also used to refer to the eardrum. *Myring-* is from the Latin word for drum.

The middle ear contains three tiny bones called ossicles, which transmit vibrations. Disorders of the ossicles are found under H74 *Other disorders of middle ear mastoid*.

The inner ear block is **H80-H83** (Diseases of inner ear). The inner ear consists of a series of canals shaped like a maze. These canals are called the **labyrinth** from the Greek work for maze. Find code H83.0 *Labyrinthitis*, which, of course, means inflammation of the labyrinth. The labyrinth contains the cochlea, a snail shaped winding tube that contains the receptor for hearing.

The first code in the inner ear block is H80 *Otosclerosis*. You know that *ot-* means
the ear. Do you remember that
sclerosis comes from the Greek
word for hard? So, otosclerosis is
hardening of the inner ear.

H90-H94 (Other disorders of ear)
is the next block of codes. Find
code H92 *Otalgia and effusion of*

> **It's all GREEK** [or Latin] **to me!**
>
> **effus(e)(ion)** – to pour out
> **labyrinth** – maze
> **myring** – the ear drum
> **-rrhea** – discharge of pus or fluid

ear. Effusion comes from the Latin word that means "to pour out." Notice that
there are three indented codes under H92. H92.0 *Otalgia*, which means ear pain,
H92.1 *Otorrhea*, which comes from the Greek for "flow" and indicates a discharge
of pus or fluid, and H92.2 *Otorrhagia*, which indicates bleeding from the ear. Go
back to Chapter 4 and check the roots for hemorrhage. Notice the similarity?

Many chapters in the ICD-10 have a block entitled Intraoperative and
postprocedural complications and disorders, not elsewhere classified. **Block H95** is
an example.

Practice your skill with these exercises.

8.1
Blanca has a hematoma on the external portion of her left ear. Which code is best?

_____ H61.121   _____ H61.112   _____ H61.122

8.2
Which of the following codes is for bilateral diffuse otitis externa?

_____ H60.23   _____ H60.313   _____ H60.323

8.3
Dr. Able's patient has acute serous otitis media of both ears (inflammation of the
middle ear). Which of these codes will you use?

_____ H65.03   _____ H65.113   _____ H65.23

8.1

H61.122 is the code for hematoma of pinna, left ear.

The other two choices were close, but some of the details were not correct. H61.121 is the code for hematoma of pinna, right ear. H61.112 is the code for acquired deformity of pinna, left ear.

8.2

The code for diffuse otitis externa of both ears is H60.313

Otitis externa is an inflammation of the external ear. Breaking it down: otitis means an inflammation in the ear, and externa further categorizes it as belonging to the external ear. ICD-10 requires you to break down diffuse otitis externa by location. In case the location is not in the doctor's notes, you must use "unspecified." You need to show right ear, left ear, bilateral or unspecified.

8.3

H65.03 is for acute serous otitis media of both ears.

Otitis media means inflammation of the middle ear. *Media* comes from Latin and means middle. Codes for the middle ear are found in the second block of this chapter, **H65-H75**.

QUICK QUIZ   *Answers in Appendix A*

_____	8.1 Endocrine, Nutritional and Metabolic Diseases	*A.*	Codes begin with A
_____	8.2 Certain Infectious and Parasitic Diseases	*B.*	Codes begin with D
_____	8.3 Diseases of the Blood and Blood-forming Organs	*C.*	Codes begin with G
_____	8.4 Diseases of the Nervous System	*D.*	Codes begin with E

8.4

The patient has developed a postauricular fistula of the right ear. Which code will you use?

_____ H70.81   _____ H70.812   _____ H70.811

8.5

Look at the list of Greek and Latin root words in Appendix B. Which of these prefixes means the ear?

_____ *Myo-*   _____ *Ot-*

_____ *Cephal-*   _____ *Kerato-*

8.6

Charles is having trouble hearing. The doctor determines he has impacted cerumen (a large amount of ear wax in both ears). Which code will you use?

_____ H61.23   _____ H61.303

_____ H61.20   _____ H61.301

8.7

In the middle ear, there are three tiny bones. Find code H74.313 and determine what these three bones are called.

_____ Ossicles   _____ Bilaterals

_____ Ankylosis   _____ Discontinuities

8.8

The patient's inner ear is hardening. A certain bone is becoming immobilized in both ears causing cochlear otosclerosis. Which of these is the best code? Hint: the clue is both ears.

_____ H80.20   _____ H80.90   _____ H80.23

8.4

H70.811 is the code for postauricular fistula of the right ear.

Postauricular means behind the pinna. Another word for pinna is auricle.
Postauricular has three word parts: *post-* which means behind; *auricul-* indicating
auricle; and *-ar* indicating this word is an adjective. H70.81 has codes indented
beneath it, so it is a category and should not be used as a code. H70.812 is for the
left ear, but our patient's problem was with the right ear.

8.5

Ot- means the ear.

Remember otitis? *Ot-* indicates the ear and *-itis* means inflammation.

8.6

H61.23 is the code for impacted cerumen of both ears.

H61.20 is not the best choice in this case because it is for unspecified ear and this
case is for both ears. Both H61.303 and H61.301 are for acquired stenosis of external
ear canal which is not our patient's condition.

8.7

The malleus, the incus and the stapes are the three ossicles (bones) found in the
middle ear.

These three bones transmit the vibrations from the ear drum to the inner ear.

8.8

H80.23 is for cochlear otosclerosis, bilateral. You can rule out H80.90 as it is for
unspecified ear and H81.23 is for vestibular neuronitis.

Otosclerosis is a disease of hardening of part of the ear. Breaking it down:
otosclerosis is made of three word parts: *ot-* indicates the ear; *scler-* means
hardening; *-osis* indicates disease.

8.9

Harold has cholesteatoma of the mastoid in his right ear. What is the correct code for this condition?

_____ H70.001   _____ H71.21   _____ H83.01

8.10

Dr. Able's patient has bilateral aural vertigo. Which of the following is the correct code?

_____ H81.393   _____ H81.31   _____ H81.313

8.11

Helga has a perforation of the tympanic membrane of her right ear. Which code will you put on the bill?

_____ H72.01   _____ H72.10   _____ H72.12

8.12

Harvey has an unspecified obstruction of his Eustachian tube in his left ear. What is the correct code for this condition?

_____ H68.112   _____ H68.102   _____ H68.112

8.13

Harley has inflammation of the labyrinth in both ears. Which of these codes will you use for this condition?

_____ H83.13   _____ H83.03   _____ H83.93

QUICK QUIZ Answers in Appendix A

_____ 8.5 Pain   **A.** -rrhea

_____ 8.6 To pour out   **B.** -algia

_____ 8.7 Discharge of pus or fluid   **C.** suppuratus

_____ 8.8 Producing pus   **D.** effuse(e)(ion)

8.9

H71.21 is the code for cholesteatoma of mastoid, right ear.

Cholesteatoma is a cyst-like sac filled with epithelial cells and cholesterol.

8.10

The code for aural vertigo in both ears is H81.313.

8.11

H72.01 is for a perforation of the tympanic membrane of the right ear.

The tympanic membrane separates the middle ear from the external ear. Tympanic is easy to remember because *tympan-* is from a Greek word that means drum. A common term for tympanic membrane is ear drum.

8.12

H68.102 *Unspecified obstruction of Eustachian tube, left ear* is the correct answer.

The Eustachian tube is also known as the auditory tube. Eustachian comes from Eustachio, in honor of the anatomist who named the auditory tube.

8.13

The code for inflammation of the labyrinth of both ears is H83.03 *Labyrinthitis, bilateral*.

The labyrinth is a series of intricate communicating canals hollowed out of the temporal bone. The labyrinth contains the cochlea, the vestibule and the semicircular canals.

QUICK QUIZ Answers in Appendix A

_____ 8.9	External ear	**A.** cerumen
_____ 8.10	Ear wax	**B.** labyrinth
_____ 8.11	Drum (as in ear drum)	**C.** auricle
_____ 8.12	Maze	**D.** tympan(o)

8.14

The rock musician complains of constant buzzing sounds in her head, both ears. This condition is called tinnitus. Select the correct code.

_____ H93.11   _____ H93.12   _____ H93.13

8.15

Which code is associated with the formation of pus?

_____ H92.01   _____ H66.41   _____ H92.21

8.16

Which code is associated with pain in the ear?

_____ H92.01   _____ H92.11   _____ H92.21

8.17

Dr. Able has a patient who has inflammation of the right ear with a fluid discharge. Which code is for fluid discharge from the ear?

_____ H92.20   _____ H92.11   _____ H92.09

8.18

A patient came to see Dr. Able with otorrhagia: bleeding from the external ear canal. Which code is used for this condition?

_____ H92.20   _____ H92.11   _____ H92.09

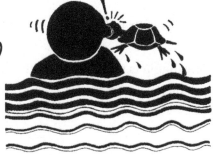

There's a code for THAT??

Turtles must be really, really dangerous.
There are codes for *Bitten by turtle* (W59.21);
Struck by turtle (W59.22); and *Other contact with turtle* (W59.29). But watch out! There's an **Excludes1** note with W59.2!

8.14

H93.13 is the code for tinnitus of both ears.

Tinnitus is a constant buzzing or ringing in the ears. Tinnitus comes from the Latin word for jingling. It may be caused by hearing loss due to natural aging (presbycusis), damage by extreme noise, or it may be a symptom of a disease, like Meniere's disease. If it is a symptom of a disease two codes may be required. We will explore this later.

8.15

H66.41 is for suppurative otitis media, unspecified, right ear.

Suppurative means producing or associated with the producing of pus.

8.16

H92.01 *Otalgia, right ear* is the code for pain in the right ear.

Otalgia is pain in the ear. You know *ot-* means ear. Did you remember that *-algia* means pain?

8.17

H92.11 is the code for otorrhea of the right ear.

Otorrhea is a flow or discharge from the ear. As you know, *ot-* means ear. *-rrhea* means a flow or discharge. The codes indented beneath H92.1 are for otorrhea and should be used according to the ear or ears involved.

8.18

H92.20 is one of the codes for otorrhagia.

Otorrhagia is bleeding from the ear. *Ot-* means ear; *-rrhgia* means bleeding. The indented codes beneath H92.2 are for otorrhagia.

You know that the suffix *-itis* means inflammation. Let's look at some words that end in *-itis*. We'll start with an easy one.

8.19

Which word describes inflammation of the mastoid process, H70?

_____ Myringitis   _____ Salpingitis

_____ Mastoiditis   _____ Labyrinthitis

8.20

Look up H83.0. What does it cover?

_____ Myringitis   _____ Salpingitis

_____ Mastoiditis   _____ Labyrinthitis

8.21

Look up H68. What does it cover?

_____ Myringitis   _____ Salpingitis

_____ Mastoiditis   _____ Labyrinthitis

8.22

Look up H73.0. What does it cover?

_____ Myringitis   _____ Salpingitis

_____ Mastoiditis   _____ Labyrinthitis

8.23

What is the block for diseases of the inner ear?

_____ **H60-H62**   _____ **H65-H75**

_____ **H80-H83**   _____ **H90-H94**

8.19

Mastoiditis is the inflammation of the mastoid process.

The two key word parts are mastoid and *–itis*.

8.20

Labyrinthitis is inflammation of the labyrinth, which is the intricate communicating canals hollowed out of the temporal bone in the inner ear.

8.21

Eustachian salpingitis is inflammation of the Eustachian tube.

Look at code H68 in your ICD-10. *Salping-* comes from the Greek word for tube. The term salpingitis is also used to describe inflammation of the fallopian tube.

8.22

Myringitis is the inflammation of the ear drum.

Myring- is from the Latin for drum. Look up myringitis in the alphabetical index. You'll find several types of myringitis listed. Once you find the term in the alphabetical index, be sure and look up the code in the tabular list and check for notes that might affect coding.

8.23

Diseases of the inner ear are in **Block H80-H83**.

This chapter contains five blocks:
>   **H60-H62** (Diseases of external ear)
>   **H65-H75** (Diseases of middle ear and mastoid)
>   **H80-H83** (Diseases of inner ear)
>   **H90-H94** (Other disorders of ear)
>   **H95** (Intraoperative and postprocedural complications and disorders of ear and mastoid process, not elsewhere classified)

8.24

Look through the chapter for diseases of the ear and mastoid process. Look at the most detailed level of the diagnoses. What level of specificity do most codes have in common?

_____ Other, non-specific

_____ Ear, mastoid process

_____ Right ear, left ear, bilateral, and unspecified ear

8.25

What is the last code in the ear and mastoid process chapter?

_____

8.26

Which block(s) have information in the Chapter-Specific Coding Guidelines?

_____ **H60-H62** (Diseases of external ear)

_____ **H65-H75** (Diseases of middle ear and mastoid)

_____ **H80-H83** (Diseases of inner ear)

_____ **H90-H94** (Other disorders of ear)

_____ All of the above

_____ None of the above

8.27

A patient presents at Dr. Able's office with ototoxic hearing loss of the left ear, H91.02. Her hearing loss is due to drug poisoning. Which of the following statements is true?

_____ The first code listed should be the hearing loss code, the drug poisoning code should be listed second

_____ The first code listed should be the drug poisoning code, the hearing loss code should be listed second

_____ Only the hearing loss should be coded

8.24

At the most detailed level, most codes are listed <u>by right ear, left ear, bilateral, unspecified ear</u>.

For example, look at code H60.33 *Swimmer's ear*, which requires one of the following additional digits.

     H60.331 *Swimmer's ear, right ear*

     H60.332 *Swimmer's ear, left ear*

     H60.333 *Swimmer's ear, bilateral*

     H60.339 *Swimmer's ear, unspecified ear*

8.25

Many blocks in the ICD-10 lump "Other" under a single code. Flip to the end of this chapter in the ICD-10 and you will find that the last code in the ear and mastoid process chapter is <u>H95.89</u> *Other postprocedural complications and disorders of the ear and mastoid process, not elsewhere classified*.

8.26

The correct answer is <u>none of the above</u>.

Some chapters have no Chapter-Specific Coding Guidelines and Chapter 8 is one of them.

 HOT TIP

Checking the Chapter-Specific Coding Guidelines can mean the difference between a correct code and an incorrect code. Smart coders make the best employees (and hopefully the best salaries).

8.27

The true statement is the middle one: <u>the first code listed should be the drug poisoning code. The hearing loss code should be listed second</u>.

Why? Because after code H91.0, the first note says "Code first poisoning due to drug or toxin, if applicable (T36-T65 with fifth or sixth character 1-4)."

QUICK QUIZ *Answers in Appendix A*

_____	8.13	Lack	A. -penia
_____	8.14	Dissolution or breaking down	B. -lytic
_____	8.15	The study of	C. -ology
_____	8.16	Abnormal flow or discharge	D. -rrhage

8.28

Dr. Able has diagnosed his patient with acoustic neuritis due to a parasitic disease. The ICD-10 code for this condition is H94.01. Which of the following statements is true?

_____ The first code listed should be the acoustic neuritis code, the parasitic disease code should be listed second

_____ The first code listed should be the parasitic disease code, the acoustic neuritis code should be listed second

_____ Only the acoustic neuritis code should be listed

8.29

Based on the doctor's notes, you code the patient with H82.3 *Vertiginous syndromes in diseases classified elsewhere, bilateral*. But you notice that the patient also has epidemic vertigo, which is code A88.1. Which is the correct way to code this?

_____ A88.1 should be coded first, and then H82.3

_____ H82.3 should be coded first, and then A88.1

_____ Only H82.3 should be coded

There's a code for THAT??

If your patient has been hit by a falling object due to an accident involving a watercraft, V91.3 is the code for that. But please, be specific! ICD-10 requires that you indicate whether the watercraft was a merchant ship, passenger ship, fishing boat, other powered watercraft, sailboat, canoe or kayak, inflatable craft, water-skis (when not on fire), other unpowered craft and, just in case, unspecified watercraft.

8.28

The true statement is <u>the first code listed should be the parasitic disease code, and the acoustic neuritis code should be listed second.</u>

How do you know? There is a **"Code first"** underlying disease note listed after code H94.0.

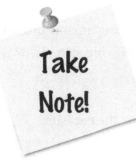

Take Note!

A lot of changes have been made since the previous version of ICD coding, which was developed in the 1970s. Even experienced coders need to learn all the new rules.

8.29

The correct way to code this diagnosis is <u>only H82.3 should be listed.</u>

If you look at the notes under H82, you might first notice a **"Code first"** underlying disease note and be tempted to code A88.1 first. However, if you look closer, you will see that A88.1 is listed in an **Excludes1** note. This means you do not use A88.1 with any of the H82 codes.

QUICK QUIZ *Answers in Appendix A*	
_____ 8.17 Endocrine, Nutritional and Metabolic Diseases	*A.* Codes begin with B
_____ 8.18 Mental, Behavioral and Neurodevelopmental Disorders	*B.* Codes begin with E
_____ 8.19 Certain Infectious and Parasitic Diseases	*C.* Codes begin with C
_____ 8.20 Neoplasms	*D.* Codes begin with F

Chapter Quiz (Answers in Appendix A)

Match the definition to the term. Some of the Greek and Latin terms from this chapter are bold.

_____ 8.1	Bleeding from the ear	A. Ot**algia**
_____ 8.2	Pain in the ear	B. Oto**rrhea**
_____ 8.3	Inflammation of the eardrum	C. Post**auricul**ar
_____ 8.4	Inflammation of the middle ear	D. **Ot**itis **media**
_____ 8.5	A flow or discharge of pus from the ear	E. **Tympan**ic membrane
_____ 8.6	Behind the pinna	F. **Ot**o**rrhagia**
_____ 8.7	Separates middle ear from external ear	G. **Myring**itis

Match the codes to the descriptors on the right. The items on the right may be used more than once.

_____ 8.8	H60.10	A. Right ear
_____ 8.9	H65.113	B. Left ear
_____ 8.10	H61.123	C. Bilateral
_____ 8.11	H68.102	D. Unspecified ear
_____ 8.12	H62.43	
_____ 8.13	H61.012	
_____ 8.14	H74.21	
_____ 8.15	H66.005	
_____ 8.16	H66.3X3	
_____ 8.17	H61.322	
_____ 8.18	H65.197	
_____ 8.19	H90.72	
_____ 8.20	H66.014	

Match the code to the block title the code is in. Each block may be used more than once.

_____ 8.21 H80.02	A. Diseases of external ear
_____ 8.22 H61.322	B. Diseases of middle ear and mastoid
_____ 8.23 H65.114	C. Diseases of inner ear
_____ 8.24 H83.02	D. Other disorders of ear
_____ 8.25 H60.323	E. Intraoperative and postprocedural complications and disorders of ear and mastoid process, NEC
_____ 8.26 H90.11	
_____ 8.27 H68.012	
_____ 8.28 H80.21	
_____ 8.29 H61.122	
_____ 8.30 H70.001	
_____ 8.31 H71.22	
_____ 8.32 H92.03	
_____ 8.33 H72.01	
_____ 8.34 H81.01	
_____ 8.35 H92.22	
_____ 8.36 H74.03	
_____ 8.37 H93.213	
_____ 8.38 H95.111	
_____ 8.39 H93.3X3	
_____ 8.40 H61.23	

9

Diseases of the Circulatory System

Now let's explore the fascinating codes covering the circulatory system. The first block is **I00-I02** (Acute rheumatic fever), followed by **I05-I09** (Chronic rheumatic heart diseases). *Acute*, from the Latin for sharp or severe, indicates a rapid onset of a condition or disease. *Chronic*, from the Greek for "over time," means that the condition has been occurring for a period of time. Rheumatic indicates that this is an inflammatory disease. As you'll begin to see, knowing about 100 of the most common of the Greek and Latin root words will make coding much easier.

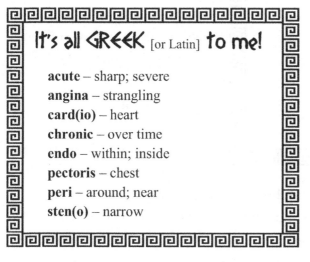

It's all GREEK [or Latin] **to me!**

acute – sharp; severe
angina – strangling
card(io) – heart
chronic – over time
endo – within; inside
pectoris – chest
peri – around; near
sten(o) – narrow

Let's start by looking at three codes: I01.0 *Acute rheumatic pericarditis*, I01.1 *Acute rheumatic endocarditis*, and I01.2 *Acute rheumatic myocarditis*. What's the difference in these three conditions? The Latin root word *Card-* means heart (you probably already knew that: think cardio workout). So, carditis is inflammation of the heart. The sac that surrounds the heart is the pericardium (*peri-* is Greek for near), so inflammation of the pericardium is pericarditis. *Endo-* is from Greek meaning within. Endocarditis, then, is inflammation of the lining within the heart. The third term, myocarditis means inflammation of the heart muscle. *Myo-*, you remember, is from the Greek word for muscle.

Now look at I06.0 *Rheumatic aortic stenosis*. Stenosis is from a Greek word for narrow. In this case, the aorta is narrowing.

Hypertension, which means high blood pressure, can lead to many complications. There is a special block for hypertensive diseases, **I10-I1A**. Notice that this block, though small, contains many **"Use additional code"** and **Excludes1** notes. Not paying attention to them can trip up even the best coders.

Locate the block for ischemic heart diseases, **I20-I25**. Ischemic comes from two Greek words: *Ische-* (to hold back), and *-emia* (blood). Ischemic heart disease is local and temporary deficiency of blood due to an obstruction of the circulation to that part of the body. Look at the first code in this block, I20 *Angina pectoris*. Angina pectoris is chest pain often due to a lack of circulation to the heart muscle.

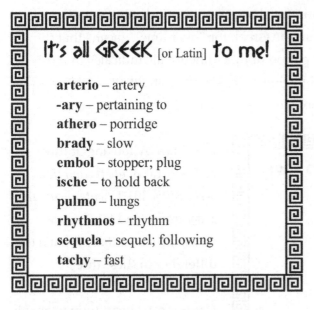

It's all GREEK [or Latin] to me!

arterio – artery
-ary – pertaining to
athero – porridge
brady – slow
embol – stopper; plug
ische – to hold back
pulmo – lungs
rhythmos – rhythm
sequela – sequel; following
tachy – fast

Find I25.1 *Atherosclerotic heart disease of native coronary artery* in your ICD-10 book. **Athero-** comes from Greek and means porridge. *Scler-*, as you learned in the last chapter, means hardening. Atherosclerosis is hardening of the artery. It is one of the most common forms of arteriosclerosis.

Pulmonary comes from the Latin word for lungs. Therefore, **Block I26-I28** (Pulmonary heart disease and diseases of pulmonary circulation) deals with conditions involving the heart and lungs. Find the first code in this block, I26 *Pulmonary embolism*. Embolism comes from a Greek word and means the blocking of a blood vessel by a foreign substance or a blood clot. Thrombus, as we learned in Chapter 4, also comes from a Greek word and also means blood clot.

Find code I47 *Paroxysmal tachycardia* and the indented codes following it. It is part of **Block I30-I52** (Other forms of heart disease). *Tachy-* is from the Greek word for fast, so tachycardia is a condition in which the heart is beating too fast. The opposite of tachycardia is bradycardia. *Brady-* comes from the Greek for slow. An irregular heartbeat is cardiac arrhythmia, for example code I49.

Cardiomyopathy is a big word, but by using our new technique we know you can decode it. *Cardio-* means the heart. In Chapter 6 you learned that *myo-* means muscle and *-pathy* means disease, therefore cardiomyopathy is a disease of the heart muscle. Look for code I42 *Cardiomyopathy.*

Block I60-I69 covers cerebrovascular diseases. You know that *cerebro-* means the brain. If you remember, *-vascular* is a Latin word that refers to blood vessels. So, cerebrovascular refers to the blood vessels of the brain.

Look at code I69 *Sequelae of cerebrovascular disease.* Read the note that follows this code. Sequelae is the plural form of the word sequela. You can remember these words by thinking of a movie sequel. The sequel is the movie that follows the original movie. In medicine, a sequela is a condition that is a consequence of a previous disease or injury.

The blood vessels that carry blood away from the heart are called arteries. Find **Block I70-I79** (Diseases of arteries, arterioles and capillaries). This block is followed by **I80-I89** (Diseases of veins, lymphatic vessels and lymph nodes, not elsewhere classified). Veins carry blood toward the heart and lymphatic vessels carry lymph toward the heart.

Are you pumped? Let's explore this chapter by practicing with some codes.

9.1
Which code is for inflammation of the heart, carditis?

_____ I51.7   _____ I51.81   _____ I51.89

9.2
Which code is for chronic adhesive pericarditis?

_____ I31   _____ I31.0   _____ I31.1

9.3
Which code is for supraventricular tachycardia?

_____ I47.1   _____ I47.2   _____ I47.9

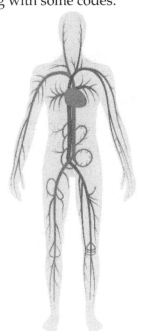

QUICK QUIZ *Answers in Appendix A*

_____ 9.1	Localized neoplasm	**A.**	Malignant
_____ 9.2	Non-cancerous	**B.**	Neoplasm
_____ 9.3	Cancerous	**C.**	Benign
_____ 9.4	Tumor or growth	**D.**	In situ

9.1

Look at code I51.89 *Other ill-defined heart diseases*. Carditis is listed below it.

Carditis is inflammation of the heart. It is made up of two word parts you already know: *card-* for heart and *-itis* for inflammation.

9.2

I31.0 is a code for chronic adhesive pericarditis, inflammation of the sac that surrounds the heart.

The pericardium is the sac that surrounds the heart. Look at the word parts. *Peri-* means surrounding or enclosing. The term *-cardium,* as you know, means the heart. *-itis* means inflammation. Put them together and you get pericarditis.

9.3

The code for supraventricular tachycardia is I47.1.

I47.2 won't work because it is for ventricular tachycardia and I47.9 isn't correct because it is for paroxysmal tachycardia. Tachycardia is an abnormally fast heartbeat. *Tachy-* means fast. *-cardia* means the heart.

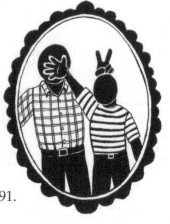

There's a code for THAT??

Yes, for real! ICD-10 has a code for conditions due to sibling rivalry. It's Z62.891.

9.4

A patient has endocarditis; the membrane that lines the inside of his heart is inflamed. Which of these codes below is a code for this condition?

_____ I33.9   _____ I40.9   _____ I67.82

9.5

What is the category for acute myocarditis?

_____ I33   _____ I40   _____ I41

9.6

Look at the Greek and Latin boxes at the beginning of this chapter. Which term means a condition following and resulting from a disease or injury? Look at I69.

_____ Ischemia   _____ Sequelae   _____ Stenosis

9.7

Irving has been diagnosed with cerebral ischemia, which is in the category for other cerebral vascular diseases, I67. Which one of these codes will you use?

_____ I67.0   _____ I67.4   _____ I67.82

9.8

Deion has rheumatic mitral stenosis with insufficiency, found in category I05, rheumatic mitral valve diseases. Which of the following codes will you use for his specific condition?

_____ I05.0   _____ I05.1   _____ I05.2

QUICK QUIZ *Answers in Appendix A*	
_____ 9.5 Tumor, swelling	*A.* -oma
_____ 9.6 Condition	*B.* -plegia
_____ 9.7 Stroke, paralysis	*C.* -osis
_____ 9.8 Refers to vision	*D.* -opia

9.4

I33.9 is one of the codes used for endocarditis.

Break the word endocarditis into its parts: *Endo-* means inside. *Card-* means the heart. *-itis* means inflammation.

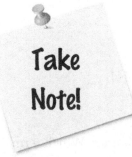

Look up endocarditis in the alphabetical index.
You will find many listings for it.
Not all listings for endocarditis are
located in this chapter of the ICD-10.

9.5

I40 is the category for myocarditis.

Myocarditis is inflammation of the heart muscle. More specifically, it is inflammation of the myocardium, the middle layer of the walls of the heart which is composed of muscles. *Myo-* means muscle. *Card-* means heart. *-itis*, as always, means inflammation.

9.6

Sequelae is used when a condition follows and is the result of an illness or injury.

9.7

I67.82 is for cerebral ischemia. Ischemia is a local and temporary deficiency of blood because of an obstruction of the circulation to that part of the body. Since ischemia can occur in many parts of the body, it is used in various places in the ICD-10.

9.8

I05.2 is for rheumatic mitral stenosis with insufficiency. Stenosis describes a narrowing or constriction of a passageway

Look up stenosis in the alphabetical index. You will see there are many situations in which stenosis occurs.

9.9

Which code indicates essential hypertension, a condition in which the patient's blood pressure is higher than normal?

_____ I10   _____ I12

_____ I11   _____ I12.0

9.10

Which code is used for angina pectoris with documented spasm?

_____ I20   _____ I20.1

_____ I20.0   _____ I20.8

9.11

Yesenia has a disease of the muscle of the heart, called dilated cardiomyopathy. What code will you use?

_____ I42   _____ I42.1

_____ I42.0   _____ I42.2

9.12

Kyle has an irregular heartbeat, cardiac arrhythmia. The doctor's notes don't specify further. Which code will you use?

_____ I49   _____ I49.8

_____ I49.40   _____ I49.9

9.13

Margarita's doctor has diagnosed her with acute embolism and thrombosis of an unspecified vein. Which code will you use?

_____ I82.3   _____ I82.90

_____ I82.891   _____ I82.91

9.9

I10 is the code for essential hypertension.

Hypertension is a condition in which the patient's blood pressure is higher than normal. *Hyper-* means overexcited, overstimulated, over, above, etc. There is an entire block of codes for hypertensive diseases (**I10-I1A**).

9.10

I20.1 is used for angina pectoris with documented spasm.

Angina pectoris, in category I20, is a term that means chest pain. *Angina* derives from the Latin for strangling and *pectoris* comes from the Latin for chest. Angina pectoris means a strangling feeling in the chest. You can't just use code I20, ICD-10 requires you to be more specific.

9.11

I42.0 is the code for dilated cardiomyopathy.

Cardiomyopathy is a disease of the heart muscle. *Cardio-* means heart. *Myo-* means muscle. *-pathy* means disease. You can find it under I42 and I43.

9.12

I49.9 is correct, the other choices are specified and I49 is the category.

An irregular heartbeat is cardiac arrhythmia. As you know, cardiac refers to the heart. Arrhythmia means irregular rhythm. *A-* = no or not and *-rrhythmia* = rhythm.

9.13

I82.90 is the only choice that has all the key factors: acute, embolism and thrombosis, and finally, unspecified vein.

Thrombosis is the formation of a blood clot inside a blood vessel which obstructs the flow of blood. Recall that embolism is the blocking of a blood vessel by a foreign substance or by a blood clot.

9.14

Mrs. Periwinkle has an inflamed superficial vein in her right leg, a condition known as phlebitis. Which code will you choose?

_____ I80.00   _____ I80.01

_____ I80.02   _____ I80.03

9.15

Mr. Dandelion has thrombophlebitis of his left iliac vein. Which code will you choose?

_____ I80.211   _____ I80.212

_____ I80.213   _____ I80.219

9.16

Miss Daisy's doctor has given her a diagnosis of atherosclerosis of native arteries of her left leg with ulceration of her calf. Which code will you use?

_____ I70.222   _____ I70.232

_____ I70.242   _____ I70.262

9.17

Chapter 9 Diseases of the Circulatory System has quite a few Chapter-Specific Coding Guidelines. Look at the guidelines for hypertensive cerebrovascular disease. According to the guidelines, which code should be listed first: I60-I69 or the appropriate hypertension code?

_____ I60-I69   _____ The appropriate hypertension code.

9.18

What is the first character of codes in the circulatory system chapter?

_____ H   _____ I   _____ J   _____ K   _____ None of the above

9.14

I80.01 is the code for phlebitis of right lower extremity.

Phlebitis is the inflammation of a vein, most commonly in the leg. Look at the word parts: *phleb-* means vein and *-itis* means inflammation.

9.15

I80.212 is the code for thrombophlebitis of the left iliac vein.

Thrombophlebitis is a blood clot in a vein and the vein is inflamed. Thrombophlebitis comes from three word parts. *Thrombo-* means thrombus (a blood clot), *phleb-* means vein, and, of course, *-itis* means inflammation.

9.16

I70.242 is the best code.

Atherosclerosis is a specific form of arteriosclerosis, the hardening of artery walls. *Athero-* means porridge and *-sclerosis* means hardening. Look at the many codes indented under I70.

9.17

The Chapter-Specific Coding Guidelines say that for hypertensive cerebrovascular disease, the appropriate code from I60-I69 should be assigned first, followed by the appropriate hypertension code.

Take Note!

Guideline a) number 4 regarding hypertensive cerebrovascular disease is a good example of how the Chapter-Specific Coding Guidelines can help you select the correct code.

9.18

Codes in Chapter 9, Diseases of the Circulatory System, begin with the letter I.

9.19

Which of the following is NOT one of the blocks in the circulatory system chapter?

_____ Acute rheumatic fever   _____ Hypertensive diseases
_____ Ischemic heart diseases   _____ Influenza and pneumonia
_____ Cerebrovascular diseases

9.20

Code I06 _Rheumatic aortic valve diseases_ is found in what block?

_____ Acute rheumatic fever   _____ Chronic rheumatic heart diseases
_____ Hypertensive diseases   _____ Ischemic heart diseases

9.21

Code I65 _Occlusion and stenosis of precerebral arteries, not resulting in cerebral infarction_ is found in what block?

_____ Hypertensive diseases   _____ Ischemic heart diseases
_____ Cerebrovascular diseases   _____ Diseases of arteries, arterioles
                                               and capillaries

9.22

Look at code I50 _Heart failure_ and read the **"Code first"** note. A patient has both left ventricular failure and rheumatic heart failure. Which should be listed first?

_____ Left ventricular failure   _____ Rheumatic heart failure

9.23

You notice that one claim has two codes, I67.1 and I72.0. Can these two codes be correctly used on the same claim?

_____ Yes   _____ No

9.19

Influenza and pneumonia is not a block in the Diseases of the Circulatory System chapter. They are found in Chapter 10, which covers the respiratory system.

Chapter 9 is divided by type of heart disease.

9.20

Chronic rheumatic heart disease includes codes I05-I09.

9.21

Cerebrovascular diseases includes codes I60-I69.

9.22

Rheumatic heart failure should be coded first.

The **"Code first"** note instructs you to list the rheumatic heart failure first, and then the left ventricular failure.

9.23

No, codes I67.1 and I72.0 cannot be used at the same time.

Why not? Because code I72.0 has an **Excludes1** note that specifically excludes code I67.1.

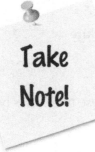

Remember, an **Excludes1** note means NOT coded here.
These codes can NOT be used together.

9.24

You notice that both I97.711 and J95.1 are coded on the same claim. Can these two codes be used on the same claim?

_____ Yes   _____ No

9.25

You see a claim that is coded with both I25.701 and I20.1 on the same claim. Can these two codes be used on the same claim?

_____ Yes   _____ No

9.26

Which block includes I02 _Rheumatic chorea_?

_____ Acute rheumatic fever   _____ Chronic rheumatic heart diseases
_____ Hypertensive diseases   _____ Ischemic heart diseases
_____ Pulmonary heart disease and diseases of pulmonary circulation

9.27

In which block will you find I25.2 _Old myocardial infarction_?

_____ Acute rheumatic fever   _____ Chronic rheumatic heart diseases
_____ Hypertensive diseases   _____ Ischemic heart diseases
_____ Pulmonary heart disease and diseases of pulmonary circulation

9.28

Which block includes I60 _Nontraumatic subarachnoid hemorrhage_?

_____ Other forms of heart disease
_____ Cerebrovascular diseases
_____ Diseases of arteries, arterioles and capillaries
_____ Diseases of veins, lymphatic vessels and lymph nodes, not elsewhere
classified

9.24

<u>Yes</u>, I97.711 and J95.1 can be coded at the same time.

Look at code I97.7. There is an **Excludes2** note for this category and J95.1 is listed. Remember, an **Excludes2** note means that the condition that is excluded (J95.1) is not part of this condition (I97.711). So, these conditions can be coded together.

9.25

<u>No</u>, I25.701 and I20.1 cannot be coded at the same time.

Why? Look at code I25.701. It has an **Excludes1** note that mentions I20.1. This means that these two codes cannot be listed at the same time.

9.26

I02 *Rheumatic chorea* is located in the <u>Acute rheumatic fever</u> block.

Acute rheumatic fever includes code I00-I02.

9.27

I25.2 *Old myocardial infarction* is located in the <u>Ischemic heart diseases</u> block.

Ischemic heart diseases includes codes I20-I25.

9.28

I60 *Nontraumatic subarachnoid hemorrhage* is located in the <u>Cerebrovascular diseases</u> block.

Cerebrovascular diseases includes codes I60-I69.

There's a code for THAT??

Did the patient have a problem while mopping? You guessed it! Y93.E5 *Activity, floor mopping and cleaning.*

Chapter Quiz (Answers in Appendix A)

Using your knowledge of Greek and Latin roots, match the definition to the word. Some of the Greek and Latin terms from this chapter are bold.

_____ 9.1	Inflammation of the heart	A. Tachy**cardia**
_____ 9.2	A local and temporary deficiency of blood because of an obstruction of circulation	B. Endo**card**itis
		C. Thrombosis
_____ 9.3	A disease of the muscle of the heart	D. Phlebitis
_____ 9.4	A condition in which the patient's blood pressure is higher than normal	E. Sequelae
		F. **Athero**sclerosis
_____ 9.5	Irregular heartbeat	G. **Card**itis
_____ 9.6	Narrowing of an orifice or passageway	H. **Ische**mia
_____ 9.7	Inflammation of sac surrounding the heart	I. Hypertension
_____ 9.8	Formation of blood clot inside a blood vessel which obstructs the flow of blood	J. Myo**card**itis
		K. Peri**card**itis
_____ 9.9	Chest pain	L. **Steno**sis
_____ 9.10	Inflammation of the membrane that lines the inside of the heart	M. **Cardio**myopathy
		N. Peri**card**ium
_____ 9.11	Inflammation of a vein	O. Angina pectoris
_____ 9.12	Abnormally fast heartbeat	P. **Card**iac ar**rhythm**ia
_____ 9.13	Hardening of an artery	Q. Acute
_____ 9.14	A condition that is following and resulting from a disease or injury	
_____ 9.15	A rapid onset of a disease or condition	
_____ 9.16	The sac that surrounds the heart	
_____ 9.17	Inflammation of the heart muscle	

Use the alphabetical index to find the code for each description.

_____ 9.18   Hypotension due to drugs

_____ 9.19   Acute nonspecific idiopathic pericarditis

_____ 9.20   Coronary atherosclerosis due to lipid rich plaque

_____ 9.21   Apraxia following nontraumatic subarachnoid
                    hemorrhage

_____ 9.22   Acute rheumatic endocarditis

_____ 9.23   Essential (primary) hypertension

_____ 9.24   Obstructive hypertrophic cardiomyopathy

_____ 9.25   Phlebitis and thrombophlebitis of other deep vessels of
                    left lower extremity

_____ 9.26   Nontraumatic subarachnoid hemorrhage from right
                    carotid siphon and bifurcation

_____ 9.27   Saddle embolus of pulmonary artery with acute cor
                    pulmonale

Indicate all appropriate notes for each code.

9.28 I09.81 _____ _____	A. **Includes**
9.29 I20.1 _____ _____ _____	B. **Excludes1**
9.30 I60.12 _____ _____ _____	C. **Excludes2**
9.31 I74.11 _____ _____ _____	D. **"Use additional code"**
9.32 I40.0 _____ _____ _____ _____	E. **"Code first"**
9.33 I70.243 _____ _____ _____	
9.34 I85.10 _____ _____ _____	
9.35 I49.01 _____ _____ _____	
9.36 I26.90 _____ _____ _____ _____	

10

Diseases of the Respiratory System

Who knew there was a medical term for the common cold? The ICD-10 code is J00 and its name is acute nasopharyngitis. *Naso-* means the nose and *pharyng-* refers to the pharynx (throat), so nasopharyngitis is inflammation of the nose and the pharynx.

The first block in this chapter includes four sinuses called the paranasal sinuses because they communicate with the nose. (Remember from Chapter 4 that the Greek prefix *para-* means near). The maxillary sinuses are located on both sides of the nose. Find code J01.0 *Acute maxillary sinusitis.* The frontal sinuses are on both sides of the forehead. Locate code J01.1 *Acute frontal sinusitis.* The ethmoid sinuses are located just above the bridge of the nose and below the frontal sinuses. Look at code J01.2 *Acute ethmoidal sinusitis.* The sphenoid sinus is in the cavity in the sphenoid bone, a large bone at the base of the skull, which sits behind the ethmoid sinus. Find code J01.3 *Acute sphenoidal sinusitis.*

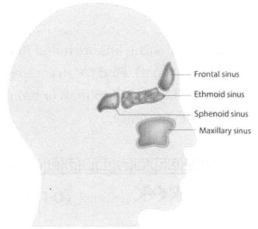

Frontal sinus
Ethmoid sinus
Sphenoid sinus
Maxillary sinus

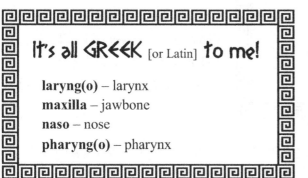

It's all GREEK [or Latin] to me!

laryng(o) – larynx
maxilla – jawbone
naso – nose
pharyng(o) – pharynx

The tonsils and adenoids are lymphatic tissue at the back of the mouth near the beginning of the pharynx. Find codes J02 *Acute pharyngitis* and J03 *Acute tonsillitis.* The larynx is located in the neck and facilitates sound production and breathing.

The epiglottis covers the larynx when swallowing. The trachea is a tube that connects the pharynx and larynx to the lungs and allows for the passage of air to the lungs. Locate code J04 *Acute laryngitis and tracheitis* in your ICD-10 code book.

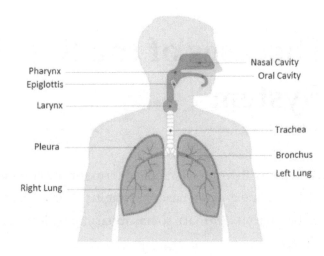

Pharynx
Epiglottis
Larynx
Pleura
Right Lung
Nasal Cavity
Oral Cavity
Trachea
Bronchus
Left Lung

Codes for influenza and pneumonia are found in **Block J09-J18**. *Pneum-* is Greek for lungs and *-ia* is Latin for disease or condition.

Bronchitis and bronchiolitis are found in **Block J20-J22** (Other acute lower respiratory infections). Find J20 *Acute bronchitis* and J21 *Acute bronchiolitis* in your ICD-10 book. The bronchi (plural) or bronchus (singular) are passageways that conduct air into the lungs.

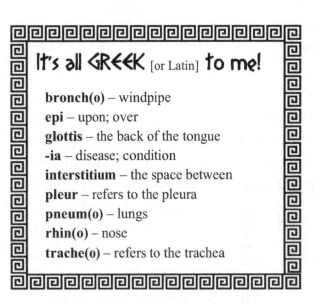

It's all GREEK [or Latin] to me!

bronch(o) – windpipe
epi – upon; over
glottis – the back of the tongue
-ia – disease; condition
interstitium – the space between
pleur – refers to the pleura
pneum(o) – lungs
rhin(o) – nose
trache(o) – refers to the trachea

Block J30-J39 covers other diseases of the upper respiratory tract. This block includes various conditions such as J31 *Chronic rhinitis, nasopharyngitis and pharyngitis.*

Chronic lower respiratory diseases are covered in **Block J40-J4A** which includes J42 *Unspecified chronic bronchitis* and J45 *Asthma.*

Conditions involving lung diseases due to external agents such as dust, gases, fumes and vapors are found in **Block J60-J70**.

The interstitium (Latin for "the space between") is all the space between body parts, cells, or tissues. **Block J80-J84** covers conditions affecting the interstitium. The pleura is a membrane that enfolds and protects the lungs. The term pleural refers to the pleura, and effusion means to pour out. Pleural effusion is an excess of fluid in the pleura. This condition can be found in **Block J90-J94** (Other diseases of the pleura).

Take Note!

Many chapters have a block for codes to use when there are complications of medical procedures that occur either during or following the procedure. An example is J95. The long name for this code is "Intraoperative and postprocedural complications and disorders of respiratory system, not elsewhere classified." For an example, locate code J95.82 Postprocedural respiratory failure.

Breathe deeply, now, and work these practice exercises.

10.1
What's another name for the common cold, code J00?

_____ Sinusitis   _____ Tonsillitis   _____ Rhinitis

10.2
Which code is for acute recurrent maxillary sinusitis?

_____ J01.01   _____ J01.11   _____ J01.21

10.3
Which code is for acute frontal sinusitis, unspecified?

_____ J01.1   _____ J01.10   _____ J01.11

10.4
Which code is the diagnosis for acute recurrent ethmoidal sinusitis?

_____ J01.2   _____ J01.20   _____ J01.21

10.1

Rhinitis is another name for the common cold.

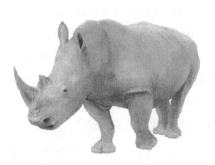

Rhin- is from the Greek for nose. *-itis*, of course, means inflammation. Rhinitis is the inflammation of the mucous lining of the nose.

10.2

The correct answer is J01.01 *Acute recurrent maxillary sinusitis.*

There are more than a dozen codes under J01. ICD-10 requires you to be specific.

10.3

The correct answer is J01.10 *Acute frontal sinusitis, unspecified.*

10.4

The correct answer is J01.21 *Acute recurrent ethmoidal sinusitis.*

The J01 codes are organized by sinus (maxillary, frontal, ethmoidal, sphenoidal, and pansinusitis, which means all sinuses). There are also codes for other and codes for unspecified. Each sinus category is further broken down into unspecified and recurrent. Therefore, you should code acute ethmoidal sinusitis, unspecified as J01.20 but acute recurrent ethmoidal sinusitis should be coded as J01.21.

QUICK QUIZ *Answers in Appendix A*

_____ 10.1 Symptoms and Signs	**A.** Codes begin with R
_____ 10.2 Congenital Malformations	**B.** Codes begin with Q
_____ 10.3 Mental and Behavioral	**C.** Codes begin with O
_____ 10.4 Pregnancy	**D.** Codes begin with F

10.5

Which is the code for acute sphenoidal sinusitis, unspecified?

_____ J01.10   _____ J01.20   _____ J01.30

10.6

June has sinusitis that is acute and unspecified. Which is the best code for her condition?

_____ J01.00   _____ J01.20   _____ J01.30
_____ J01.40   _____ J01.80   _____ J01.90

10.7

Mr. Garcia has streptococcal pharyngitis, inflammation of the tube that extends from the back of the nose to the esophagus. Which code will you select?

_____ J02.0   _____ J02.8   _____ J02.9

10.8

Holly has acute laryngitis, inflammation of the body part that opens at the base of the tongue and extends down to the trachea. Which of these is the best code?

_____ J04.0   _____ J04.1   _____ J04.2

10.9

Richard has been diagnosed with acute streptococcal tonsillitis. It is recurrent. What code will you use?

_____ J03   _____ J03.0   _____ J03.00
_____ J03.01   _____ J03.8   _____ J03.91

10.5

The correct answer is <u>J01.30</u> *Acute sphenoidal sinusitis, unspecified.*

10.6

<u>J01.90</u> *Acute sinusitis, unspecified* is the best choice.

10.7

<u>J02.0</u> is the code for streptococcal pharyngitis.

The pharynx is a passage for both the respiratory and the digestive systems. *Pharyng-* = pharynx and *-itis* = inflammation.

10.8

<u>J04.0</u> is the code for acute laryngitis.

A common name for the larynx is voice box. If you have an inflamed voice box you may temporarily lose your voice. *Laryng-* = larynx and *-itis* = inflammation.

10.9

The best code is <u>J03.01</u> *Acute recurrent streptococcal tonsillitis.*

An inflammation of the tonsils is called tonsillitis. Be sure you choose the most detailed code that matches the condition. In this case, the keys are acute, streptococcal and recurrent.

QUICK QUIZ *Answers in Appendix A*

_____ 10.5 Nervous System	*A.*	Codes begin with K
_____ 10.6 Digestive System	*B.*	Codes begin with L
_____ 10.7 Ear and Mastoid Process	*C.*	Codes begin with H
_____ 10.8 Skin and Subcutaneous Tissue	*D.*	Codes begin with G

10.10

Alvin's doctor has diagnosed him with bronchitis. He notes in the chart that it is acute and due to streptococcus. Which code will you use?

_____ J20.0   _____ J20.1   _____ J20.2

10.11

Miriam's doctor has diagnosed her with acute tracheitis without obstruction. Which code will you choose?

_____ J04.1   _____ J04.10   _____ J04.11

10.12

Which code can you use for pleural effusion?

_____ J90   _____ J91   _____ J92

10.13

Alexandria has been diagnosed with acute epiglottitis with obstruction, an inflammation of the epiglottis. Which code will you use?

_____ J05.1   _____ J05.10   _____ J05.11

10.14

Which of these codes is used for a choanal polyp of the nasal cavity?

_____ J33   _____ J33.0   _____ J33.8

10.15

Donald comes in with pharyngitis, an acute sore throat. What's the best code for this condition?

_____ J01.8   _____ J02.9   _____ J03.00

10.10

J20.2 is the code for acute bronchitis due to streptococcus.

The bronchi (bronchus) are passageways that conduct air into the lungs. *Bronch-* = bronchi and *-itis* = inflammation.

10.11

J04.10 is the code for acute tracheitis without obstruction.

The trachea is a tube that connects the pharynx and larynx to the lungs and allows for the passage of air to the lungs. *Trache-* = trachea and *-itis* = inflammation.

10.12

J90 is used for pleural effusion. Remember, do not use codes if there are codes indented beneath them, so J91 is not a good answer.

The pleura enfold, or surround, both lungs. You will see diagnoses involving the pleura in **Block J90-J94** (Other diseases of the pleura).

10.13

J05.11 *Acute epiglottitis with obstruction* is the best choice.

The epiglottis is the structure that covers the entrance of the larynx when we swallow and *-itis* means inflammation.

10.14

J33.0 is the best choice.

Why? Indented beneath code J33.0 is a list of conditions included in this code and choanal polyp is one of the conditions listed.

10.15

J02.9 is the code for pharyngitis, inflammation of the pharynx.

Check out code J02.9 and read the list of conditions under it.

10.16

Gary has acute nasopharyngitis. Which code will you use for this condition?

_____ J03.81   _____ J01.20   _____ J00

10.17

Which word part is the Greek word for lungs?

_____ *Pneumo-*   _____ *Tracheo-*
_____ *Broncho-*   _____ *Pharyngo-*

10.18

What is the first block of codes in the respiratory system chapter?

_____ Lung diseases due to external agents
_____ Chronic lower respiratory diseases
_____ Acute upper respiratory infections
_____ Influenza and pneumonia

10.19

According to the **Excludes2** note at the beginning of this chapter in the ICD-10, is it acceptable for two of the following codes to be used on the same bill?

An infectious and parasitic disease in the range A00-B99
One of the respiratory system codes in the range J00-J99

_____ Yes   _____ No

QUICK QUIZ *Answers in Appendix A*	
_____ 10.9 Used as a placeholder character	*A.* The letter X
_____ 10.10 NOS meaning	*B.* Three
_____ 10.11 The minimum number of characters in a code	*C.* Seven
_____ 10.12 The maximum number of characters in a code	*D.* Unspecified

10.16

J00 is the code for acute nasopharyngitis [common cold].

Nasopharyngitis describes an inflammation of the nasopharynx, the pharynx and the nose. The term nasopharyngitis combines *naso-* (nose) with *pharyng-* (throat).

10.17

Pneumo- is the Greek word for lung.

Often the name for a disease of the lung will begin with this root word. Pneumonia, pneumonitis and pneumoconiosis are a few examples.

10.18

Acute upper respiratory infections is the first block in the respiratory system chapter.

The codes in this block, **J00-J06**, consist of respiratory infections relating to the nose and pharynx (nasopharyngitis), sinus (sinusitis), pharynx (pharyngitis), tonsils (tonsillitis), larynx (laryngitis), trachea (tracheitis), and epiglottis (epiglottitis).

10.19

Yes, it is ok to bill two of the conditions at the same time.

Why? Because an **Excludes2** note means that the excluded condition is not part of the current condition, and that both conditions can be coded on the same claim.

There's a code for THAT??

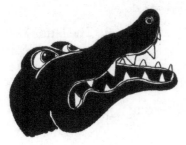

Sadly, there is a code for alligator injuries. But ICD-10 demands specifics!
Pay attention how you code it. Choices are Bitten by (W58.01), Struck by (W58.02), Crushed by (W58.03) and Other contact with (W58.09).

10.20

According to the Chapter-Specific Coding Guidelines for Chapter 10, regarding acute exacerbation of chronic obstructive bronchitis and asthma, which of the following is a true statement?

_____ An acute exacerbation is a worsening of a chronic condition
_____ A chronic exacerbation is a worsening of an acute condition
_____ Acute conditions should always be coded as primary

10.21

Look at code J01.01. What condition does this code cover?

_____ Acute maxillary sinusitis, unspecified
_____ Acute recurrent maxillary sinusitis
_____ Acute frontal sinusitis, unspecified
_____ Acute recurrent frontal sinusitis

10.22

Let's look again at code J01. Which of the following code pairs is allowed?

_____ J01.20 and J32.9   _____ J01.20 and J32.8

10.23

Maria has an acute sore throat, which Dr. Able diagnosed as streptococcal pharyngitis. Which of the following codes is an appropriate code for her condition?

_____ J00   _____ J01.41   _____ J02.0   _____ J03.8

10.24

Tommy keeps getting streptococcal tonsillitis. What is the best code for his condition?

_____ J03   _____ J03.00   _____ J03.01   _____ J03.81

10.20

The true statement is: <u>an acute exacerbation is a worsening of a chronic condition</u>. Exacerbation means worsening.

10.21

J01.01 is for *Acute recurrent maxillary sinusitis*.

Remember that the J01 codes are divided by sinus: maxillary, frontal, ethmoidal, sphenoidal and pansinusitis. There are several subcategories under J01 and several indented codes. They include "other" (J01.8) and "unspecified" (J01.9).

10.22

The code pair <u>J01.20 and J32.8</u> is allowed.

Why? Because the **Excludes2** note with J01 mentions code J32.8. This means that it is ok to use these two codes together. There is an **Excludes1** note that lists code J32.9, which means these two codes can NOT be used together.

10.23

The correct diagnosis for an acute sore throat is <u>J02.0</u>.

How so? J02.0 is for *Streptococcal pharyngitis*. There's even an **Includes** note under J02 that says "acute sore throat."

10.24

The description for <u>J03.01</u> is *Acute recurrent streptococcal tonsillitis*.

This is an example of choosing the most descriptive code. It's true that J03 *Acute tonsillitis* is what Tommy has, but it is not the most descriptive code for his condition. J03.01 more specifically describes his condition because it keeps recurring (recurrent). Also, there was no mention of it being due to "other specified organisms," so J03.81 is not the best choice.

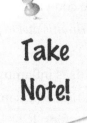

It's important to pay attention to acute vs. chronic.
Take Note!
An acute condition usually has a rapid onset and is short lived. Chronic indicates a condition that persists over time.

10.25

Sammy Sneazalot has allergic rhinitis due to pollen. At certain times of the year he really suffers from his allergies. What is the correct code for this condition?

_____ J30   _____ J30.1   _____ J30.2   _____ J30.8

10.26

Romeo comes to the doctor's office with bronchitis. The condition is acute and is the result of rhinovirus. What is the correct code for this?

_____ J20.6   _____ J20.7   _____ J31.0   _____ J41.0

10.27

Juliet has asthma, which is moderate but persistent. It is uncomplicated. Complete the code that describes this condition.

J_____

10.28

Complete the code. The patient has pulmonary edema, acute.

J_____

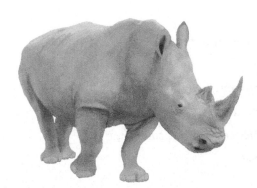

10.25

The most descriptive code for Sammy's case is J30.1 *Allergic rhinitis due to pollen.*

You know that rhinitis is inflammation of the nose. Allergic rhinitis is inflammation of the nose due to allergies. ICD-10 requires specificity when coding for allergy, in this case, its allergic rhinitis due to pollen.

10.26

The description for J20.6 is *Acute bronchitis due to rhinovirus.* Bronchitis is inflammation of the bronchial tubes.

10.27

The description for J45.40 is *Moderate persistent asthma, uncomplicated.*

How did you look up the code? You knew it began with J; did you look through all the J codes until you found asthma? Or, did you look up asthma in the alphabetical index and then look under asthma for moderate persistent? Either way will work, but it might be faster to use the alphabetical index. Remember, if you do start with the alphabetical index, you must always check the chapter listing for notes.

10.28

The description for J81.0 is *Acute pulmonary edema.*

Edema comes from a Greek word and means swelling. In this case the swelling is in the lungs (pulmonary tells you this). Did you look up edema in the alphabetical index? Under edema, you will find lung, and then you will see acute.

There's a code for THAT??

If the patient was riding his donkey and collided with a streetcar, use code V80.730 *Animal-rider injured in collision with streetcar.* However, if the patient was in a wagon being pulled by a donkey, use code V80.731 *Occupant of animal-drawn vehicle injured in collision with streetcar.*

Chapter Quiz (Answers in Appendix A)

Using your knowledge of Greek and Latin roots, match the definition to the medical word part.

_____ 10.1 Jawbone		A. rhin(o)
_____ 10.2 Lungs		B. -ia
_____ 10.3 Nose		C. maxilla
_____ 10.4 Upon; over		D. bronch
_____ 10.5 Windpipe		E. epi
_____ 10.6 Disease; condition		F. pneum(o)

Fill in the blank with the appropriate word from this list: acute, chronic, intermittent or persistent

10.7 J45.22 Mild _____ asthma with status asthmaticus

10.8 J01.00 _____ maxillary sinusitis, unspecified

10.9 J31.0 _____ rhinitis

10.10 J04.2 _____ laryngotracheitis

10.11 J41.1 Mucopurulent _____ bronchitis

10.12 J45.50 Severe _____ asthma, uncomplicated

10.13 J02.8 _____ pharyngitis due to other specified organisms

10.14 J32.2 _____ ethmoidal sinusitis

10.15 J20.7 _____ bronchitis due to echovirus

10.16 J80 _____ respiratory distress syndrome

10.17 J70.3 _____ drug-induced interstitial lung disorders

Match the code to the block title the code is in.

_____ 10.18 J67.0	A.	Acute upper respiratory infections
_____ 10.19 J20.2	B.	Influenza and pneumonia
_____ 10.20 J95.830	C.	Other acute lower respiratory infections
_____ 10.21 J45.21	D.	Other diseases of upper respiratory tract
_____ 10.22 J03.01	E.	Chronic lower respiratory diseases
_____ 10.23 J98.01	F.	Lung diseases due to external agents
_____ 10.24 J84.114	G.	Other respiratory diseases principally affecting the interstitium
_____ 10.25 J93.12	H.	Suppurative and necrotic conditions of the lower respiratory tract
_____ 10.26 J86.0	I.	Other diseases of the pleura
_____ 10.27 J38.7	J.	Interoperative and postprocedural complications and disorders of respiratory system, not elsewhere classified
_____ 10.28 J10.81	K.	Other diseases of the respiratory system

Indicate all appropriate notes for each code.

10.29 J98.11 _____ _____ _____	A.	**Includes**
10.30 J20.6 _____ _____ _____ _____	B.	**Excludes1**
10.31 J01.01 _____ _____ _____ _____	C.	**Excludes2**
10.32 J18.0 _____ _____ _____ _____	D.	**"Use additional code"**
10.33 J02.8 _____ _____ _____ _____	E.	**"Code first"**
10.34 J35.1 _____ _____ _____		
10.35 J32.3 _____ _____ _____		
10.36 J68.1 _____ _____ _____ _____		

Half-Time Review

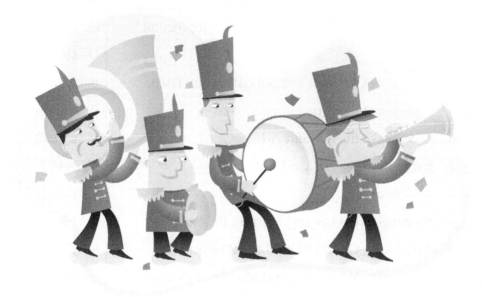

Congratulations! You've made it to the midway point. Take a moment to relax and pat yourself on the back. But not hard enough to cause S32. Or, reward yourself with an ice cream sundae (unless it would cause E73).

When you're ready, take a deep breath (but don't have an S27.309) and forge ahead to the matching review exercises by using your ICD-10 book. The answers are in Appendix A.

Half-time Review

Find the title of the chapter in which the code appears.

_____ 1. Diseases of the Musculoskeletal System	A. O77.1
_____ 2. Certain Infectious and Parasitic Diseases	B. K63.1
_____ 3. Mental, Behavioral, and Neurodevelopmental disorders	C. G37.2
	D. H02.126
_____ 4. Diseases of the Skin and Subcutaneous Tissue	E. J63.2
_____ 5. Diseases of the Circulatory System	F. M06.061
_____ 6. Diseases of the Eye and Adnexa	G. L89.42
_____ 7. External Causes of Morbidity	H. N44.2
_____ 8. Neoplasms	I. D59.2
_____ 9. Diseases of the Ear and Mastoid Process	J. F50.00
_____ 10. Pregnancy, Childbirth and the Puerperium	K. E11.311
_____ 11. Endocrine, Nutritional and Metabolic Diseases	L. H60.511
_____ 12. Diseases of the Digestive System	M. I23.3
_____ 13. Diseases of the Nervous System	N. A82.1
_____ 14. Diseases of the Blood	O. Y62.0
_____ 15. Diseases of the Respiratory System	P. C44.622
_____ 16. Diseases of the Genitourinary System	

Match the chapter to the first letter(s) of its codes.
NOTE: use H twice!

_____ 17. Circulatory System	A. Codes begin with A or B
_____ 18. Digestive System	C. Codes begin with C or D
_____ 19. Mental and Behavioral	D. Codes begin with D
_____ 20. Factors Influencing Health	E. Codes begin with E
_____ 21. Eye and Adnexa	F. Codes begin with F
_____ 22. Symptoms and Signs	G. Codes begin with G
_____ 23. Neoplasms	H. Codes begin with H
_____ 24. Respiratory System	H. Codes begin with H
_____ 25. Nervous System	I. Codes begin with I
_____ 26. Skin and Subcutaneous Tissue	J. Codes begin with J
_____ 27. Pregnancy	K. Codes begin with K
_____ 28. Congenital Malformations	L. Codes begin with L
_____ 29. Certain Infectious Diseases	M. Codes begin with M
_____ 30. Ear and Mastoid Process	N. Codes begin with N
_____ 31. Injuries or Poisoning	O. Codes begin with O
_____ 32. Diseases of the Blood	P. Codes begin with P
_____ 33. The Perinatal Period	Q. Codes begin with Q
_____ 34. Endocrine Diseases	R. Codes begin with R
_____ 35. Genitourinary System	S. Codes begin with S or T
_____ 36. Musculoskeletal System	Z. Codes begin with Z

Match the meanings to the Greek or Latin word parts.

_____ 37. Around; near	A. poly
_____ 38. Tumor; swelling	B. hemi
_____ 39. Pain	C. -osis
_____ 40. Inflammation	D. cephal(o)
_____ 41. Good; non-cancerous	E. -pathy
_____ 42. Sequel; following	F. -emia
_____ 43. Sharp; severe	G. scler
_____ 44. Half	H. -itis
_____ 45. Medium; middle	I. hyper
_____ 46. Many	J. -algia
_____ 47. No; not	K. benign
_____ 48. Disease; disorder	L. -penia
_____ 49. Blood	M. -oma
_____ 50. Condition	N. media
_____ 51. Abnormal flow or discharge	O. a(n)
_____ 52. Head; brain	P. sequela
_____ 53. Overactive; excessive	Q. acute
_____ 54. Muscle	R. peri
_____ 55. Lack	S. -rrhage
_____ 56. Hard	T. myo

Match the codes to the descriptions.

_____ 57.	C05.1	A. Drug-induced autoimmune hemolytic anemia
_____ 58.	F07.81	B. Conn's syndrome
_____ 59.	A92.31	C. Multifocal motor neuropathy
_____ 60.	I65.22	D. Recurrent pterygium of left eye
_____ 61.	G61.82	E. Hepatitis A without hepatic coma
_____ 62.	J85.1	F. Acute recurrent ethmoidal sinusitis
_____ 63.	E26.01	G. Tuberculosis of lung
_____ 64.	A15.0	H. Cochlear otosclerosis, bilateral
_____ 65.	H11.062	I. Malignant neoplasm of soft palate
_____ 66.	D59.0	J. Neoplasm of uncertain behavior of right ovary
_____ 67.	J01.21	K. Abscess of lung with pneumonia
_____ 68.	D39.11	L. Streptococcal meningitis
_____ 69.	I69.321	M. Dysphasia following cerebral infarction
_____ 70.	G00.2	N. Postconcussional syndrome
_____ 71.	B15.9	O. West Nile virus infection with encephalitis
_____ 72.	H80.23	P. Occlusion and stenosis of left carotid artery

Complete the following matching exercises.

_____ 73. Another code should be used, but does not specify which code should be first	A. **Includes**
_____ 74. The underlying condition should be coded first	B. **Excludes1**
_____ 75. Example of content in a category	C. **Excludes2**
_____ 76. You must use a different code, but can be used at the same time	D. **"Code also"**
_____ 77. The codes should never be used at the same time	E. Etiology/manifestation

Indicate all appropriate notes for each code.

78. H02.011 _____ _____	A. **Includes**
79. D77 _____ _____ _____	B. **Excludes1**
80. C03.1 _____ _____ _____	C. **Excludes2**
81. I30.1 _____ _____ _____ _____	D. **"Use additional code"**
82. A37.90 _____ _____ _____ _____	E. **"Code first"**
83. G21.2 _____ _____ _____	
84. E08.22 _____ _____ _____	
85. J95.62 _____ _____ _____	
86. F84.2 _____ _____ _____	
87. H81.393 _____ _____	
88. B67.31 _____ _____ _____ _____	
89. G80.3 _____ _____	
90. D69.42 _____ _____ _____	

11

Diseases of the Digestive System

Now that you've digested the first half of the book (hopefully without K30), let's tackle some of the body parts, terms and codes in the digestive system chapter. Using your knowledge of some key Greek and Latin base words, let's figure out the first code, K00.0 *Anodontia*. Remember the prefix *A(n)-*? It means no or not. The Greek root word for tooth is *–odont* and *–ia* is a condition. Therefore, anodontia translates to the condition of having no teeth or the absence of one or more teeth.

Now look at code K05.0 *Acute gingivitis*. You already know that *-itis* means inflammation. *Gingiva-* in Greek means gums, and as we learned in Chapter 10, acute means a single episode. So, acute gingivitis is a non-recurring inflammation of the gums.

Stoma- is the Greek word for mouth. Find K12 *Stomatitis and related lesions*. Stomatitis is inflammation of the mouth. If *glossa-* means tongue and *-dynia* means pain, then code K14.6 *Glossodynia* is a painful tongue.

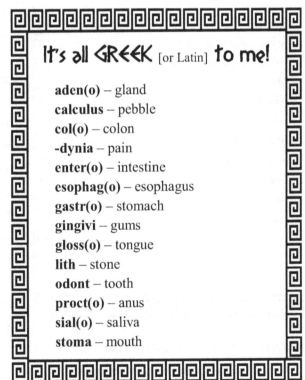

It's all GREEK [or Latin] to me!

aden(o) – gland
calculus – pebble
col(o) – colon
-dynia – pain
enter(o) – intestine
esophag(o) – esophagus
gastr(o) – stomach
gingivi – gums
gloss(o) – tongue
lith – stone
odont – tooth
proct(o) – anus
sial(o) – saliva
stoma – mouth

Moving to the second block, **K20-K31** (Diseases of esophagus, stomach and duodenum), find code K21 *Gastro-esophageal reflux disease*. Esophageal is from *esophagi-*, the Greek word for esophagus (the passage between the mouth and the stomach), and *gastro-* is Greek for stomach. So, a gastro-esophageal disease affects both the stomach and the esophagus.

Find code K29 *Gastritis and duodenitis*. Gastritis is inflammation of the stomach and duodenitis is inflammation of the duodenum.

In **Block K50-K52** you find noninfective enteritis and colitis. In medicine, the prefix *entero-* refers to the small intestine and *col-* is the root word for colon, or large intestine. Therefore, enteritis is inflammation of the small intestine, and colitis is inflammation of the colon. Find code K51.212 *Ulcerative (chronic) proctitis with intestinal obstruction*. **Proct-** is Greek for the anus, so proctitis is inflammation of the anus.

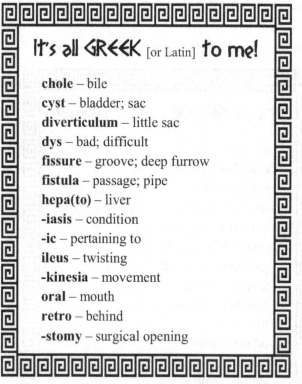

It's all GREEK [or Latin] to me!

chole – bile
cyst – bladder; sac
diverticulum – little sac
dys – bad; difficult
fissure – groove; deep furrow
fistula – passage; pipe
hepa(to) – liver
-iasis – condition
-ic – pertaining to
ileus – twisting
-kinesia – movement
oral – mouth
retro – behind
-stomy – surgical opening

You'll note a variety of other conditions involving the intestines in **Block K55-K64**. For example, find code K57.12 *Diverticulitis of small intestine without perforation or abscess without bleeding*. **Diverticula** are little sacs. Find code K60 *Fissure and fistula of anal and rectal regions*. In medicine, a *fissure* is a deep furrow, and a *fistula* is an abnormal passage connecting two body parts.

Diseases of peritoneum and retroperitoneum (**K65-K68**) is the next block. The peritoneum is the membrane that surrounds the organs in the abdomen. The term *retro-* means behind, so retroperitoneum means behind the peritoneum.

Hepat- is the Greek word for liver. **Block K70-K77** covers diseases of the liver.

Look at K80 *Cholelithiasis*, the first code in **Block K80-K87** (Disorders of gallbladder, biliary tract and pancreas). Let's break cholelithiasis into its parts. *Chole-* is bile (which is stored in the gallbladder), *lith-* means stone and *-iasis* means condition. So, cholelithiasis is the condition of having stones in the gallbladder, in casual terms, gallstones.

Now let's break down K81 *Cholecystitis*. *Chole-* (bile), plus *cyst-* (bladder) plus *-itis* (inflammation) add up to inflammation of the gallbladder.

We've chewed on some information, now let's try some exercises.

11.1

The first code in this chapter is for conditions of what body part?

_____ Teeth   _____ Gums
_____ Salivary glands   _____ Lips

11.2

Marge has a diagnosis of K05.00. This code involves what body part?

_____ Teeth   _____ Gums
_____ Salivary glands   _____ Lips

11.3

K11 covers conditions of what body part? Find this code in your ICD-10.

_____ Teeth   _____ Gums
_____ Salivary glands   _____ Lips

11.4

Homer was diagnosed with K13.0. What body part is involved?

_____ Teeth   _____ Gums
_____ Salivary glands   _____ Lips

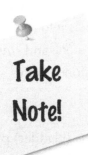

Take Note!

Did you notice that in the Greek and Latin box at the beginning of this chapter there are two terms that mean sac? *Cyst-* is from Greek and *diverticulum* is from Latin. *Diverticula* are little sacs that pouch out of an organ. Conditions that involve *diveritula* can also be found in other chapters of the ICD-10.

11.1

The first code in this chapter is for the <u>teeth</u>.

The very first set of codes in the digestive system chapter is K00 *Disorders of tooth development and eruption.*

11.2

K05.00 is for the <u>gums</u>.

They are part of the first block of codes **K00-K14** (Diseases of oral cavity and salivary glands). Look at code K05 *Gingivitis and periodontal diseases.* The root word *gingivi-* and the medical term periodontal both refer to the gums.

11.3

K11 is for *Diseases of <u>salivary glands</u>.*

They also are part of the first block of codes **K00-K14** (Diseases of oral cavity and salivary glands).

11.4

K13.0 is for *Diseases of <u>lips</u>.*

Codes for the lips are part of the first block **K00-K14** (Diseases of oral cavity and salivary glands).

11.5

Find K14.0 in your book. To what body part does this code relate?

_____ Tongue   _____ Esophagus

_____ Stomach   _____ Duodenum

11.6

What body part is involved in code K20 in your ICD-10 book?

_____ Tongue   _____ Esophagus   _____ Stomach   _____ Appendix

11.7

K29.0 covers what body part?

_____ Tongue   _____ Duodenum   _____ Stomach   _____ Appendix

11.8

What body part is involved in code K29.80?

_____ Tongue   _____ Duodenum   _____ Stomach   _____ Appendix

11.9

Which one of the following body parts is mentioned in K35.30?

_____ Tongue   _____ Duodenum   _____ Stomach   _____ Appendix

---

QUICK QUIZ _Answers in Appendix A_

_____ 11.1 Condition		**A.** -paresis
_____ 11.2 Inflammation		**B.** -ism
_____ 11.3 Muscular weakness		**C.** -pathy
_____ 11.4 Disease or disorder		**D.** -itis

11.5

K14.0 is for the <u>tongue</u>.

The tongue is part of the first block of
codes **K00-K14** (Diseases of oral cavity
and salivary glands). Code K14.0 is for
Glossitis. **Gloss-** is Greek for the tongue,
so glossitis is inflammation of the
tongue.

11.6

The <u>esophagus</u> is the body part
mentioned in K20.

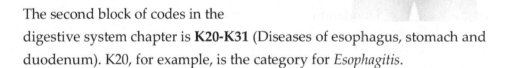

The second block of codes in the
digestive system chapter is **K20-K31** (Diseases of esophagus, stomach and
duodenum). K20, for example, is the category for *Esophagitis*.

11.7

K29.0 covers the <u>stomach</u>.

The description for K29.0 is *Acute gastritis*. **Gastr-** is the prefix for stomach.
Gastritis is inflammation of the stomach.

11.8

The <u>duodenum</u> is mentioned in K29.80.

The second block of codes in the digestive system chapter contains K29.8
Duodenitis. This is inflammation of the duodenum.

11.9

The <u>appendix</u> is mentioned in K35.30.

The appendix has its own block of codes: **K35-K38** (Diseases of appendix). You'll
find K35.30 *Acute appendicitis with localized peritonitis* here.

11.10

Bert has a diagnosis of K44.0. Which body part is being diagnosed?

_____ Diaphragm   _____ Gallbladder

_____ Peritoneum   _____ Liver

11.11

Ernie has a diagnosis of K51.913. Something is going on in which body part?

_____ Gallbladder   _____ Intestines

_____ Peritoneum   _____ Liver

11.12

Which body part can be found in **Block K65-K68**?

_____ Diaphragm   _____ Intestines   _____ Peritoneum   _____ Liver

11.13

Which body part can be found in **Block K70-K77**?

_____ Diaphragm   _____ Intestines   _____ Gallbladder   _____ Liver

11.14

Which body part can be found in **Block K80-K87**?

_____ Gallbladder   _____ Intestines   _____ Peritoneum   _____ Liver

---

QUICK QUIZ *Answers in Appendix A*

_____ 11.5 Musculoskeletal system   *A.* Codes begin with O

_____ 11.6 Pregnancy and childbirth   *B.* Codes begin with P

_____ 11.7 Perinatal period   *C.* Codes begin with M

_____ 11.8 Mental and behavioral   *D.* Codes begin with F

11.10

K44.0 *Diaphragmatic hernia with obstruction, without gangrene* is a condition of the diaphragm.

There is an entire block dedicated to hernia: **K40-K46.**

11.11

K51.913 is about the intestines.

The description of K51.913 is *Ulcerative colitis, unspecified with fistula.* The prefix *col-* refers to the colon (the large intestine). A fistula is an abnormal passage that connects two body parts. Notice there are two blocks of codes for the intestines: **K50-K52** (Noninfective enteritis and colitis) and **K55-K64** (Other diseases of intestines).

11.12

Block K65-K68 is diseases of peritoneum and retroperitoneum.

The peritoneum is a membrane that lines the abdominal cavity and retroperitoneum means behind the peritoneum.

11.13

Block K70-K77 is diseases of liver.

For an example, find code K74.1 *Hepatic sclerosis.* Remember sclerosis? It means hardening.

11.14

The gallbladder is found in **Block K80-K87.**

In this block, take a look at codes K80, K81, K82, and K83 and you'll notice several descriptions with the prefix *chole-*, such as K80 *Cholelithiasis.* This prefix means bile, and the word part *lith-* is Greek for stones.

11.15

Billy Joe's claim shows a diagnosis of K51.211. To what body part is K51.211 referring?

_____ Pancreas   _____ Anus   _____ Appendix   _____ Liver

11.16

Larissa's gums are inflamed, a condition known as gingivitis. Her chart indicates chronic, non-plaque induced. Which code will you select?

_____ K05.00   _____ K05.10
_____ K05.01   _____ K05.11

11.17

Samuel has chronic, generalized, moderate periodontitis. Which code will you use?

_____ K05.212   _____ K05.312
_____ K05.222   _____ K05.322

11.18

Mr. Goldwyn has sialolithiasis, calcified stones in one of his salivary glands. Which code will you use for this condition?

_____ K11.21   _____ K11.0
_____ K11.5   _____ K11.8

11.19

Kelly Sue has an inflammation of her parotid salivary gland. The doctor diagnosed it as acute sialoadenitis. Which code will you use for this condition?

_____ K11.20   _____ K11.22
_____ K11.21   _____ K11.23

11.15

<u>K51.211</u> *Ulcerative (chronic) proctitis with rectal bleeding* is referring to the anus.

The prefix *proct-* means anus.

11.16

Gingivitis is inflammation of the gums. The best answer is <u>K05.11</u>.

Gingivi- means the gums. Category K05 covers gingivitis and periodontal diseases.

11.17

<u>K05.322</u> is for chronic periodontitis, generalized, moderate. As you can see, ICD-10 requires very specific details, so keep scrolling down until you discover the most complete code.

Periodontitis is inflammation of the bone and gums that surround the tooth. *Peri-* means surrounding or near. *Odont-* means tooth.

11.18

The description for <u>K11.5</u> is sialolithiasis, so it is the best choice.

Sialolithiasis means calcified stones in a salivary gland. *Sialo-* is Greek for saliva and is the root word for salivary glands. In medicine, *lith-* means stones formed in the body. *-iasis* means condition. Many people think of kidney stones and gallstones but other organs and glands can form stones.

11.19

<u>K11.21</u> is for acute sialoadenitis. Be careful to watch for acute vs chronic in the diagnosis. K11.23 is for chronic sialoadenitis, so that wouldn't work in this case.

Sialoadenitis is the inflammation of a salivary gland. According to your Greek and Latin chart, *sialo-* = saliva, *adeno-* is Greek for gland, and *-itis* is inflammation. The word is easy once you break it down!

11.20

Which of these codes is for atrophy of the salivary gland?

_____ K11.0   _____ K11.3
_____ K11.1   _____ K11.4

11.21

Which of these codes is for a condition called hypertrophy?

_____ K11.0   _____ K11.3
_____ K11.1   _____ K11.4

11.22

Which of these codes is correct for oral mucositis (ulcerative) due to radiation?

_____ K12.30   _____ K12.31
_____ K12.32   _____ K12.33

11.23

One of Dr. Wellbeing's patients has ulcerative stomatitis, which is inflammation of the mouth. Which code will you use for this condition?

_____ K12.   _____ K12.0
_____ K12.1   _____ K12.30

11.24

Gabby has been diagnosed with glossitis, which is inflammation of the tongue. The doctor's notes don't specify further. What code will you use?

_____ K14   _____ K14.6
_____ K14.0   _____ K14.8

11.20

K11.0 is the best answer.

Atrophy is a condition in which a body part is wasting away. It is sometimes due to the degeneration of the cells.

11.21

K11.1 *Hypertrophy of salivary gland* is the best answer.

Hypertrophy is the medical term used when a body part is enlarging due to an increase in the size of the cells that make up the body part.

11.22

The code for oral mucositis (ulcerative) due to radiation is K12.33.

Mucositis is inflammation of mucous membranes. It usually occurs in the digestive tract, but it can also be oral (*oral* comes from the Latin word for mouth).

11.23

K12.1 is for other forms of stomatitis. Did you notice ulcerative stomatitis listed beneath K12.1?

Stomatitis is inflammation of the mouth. As you know, *oral* is the Latin word for mouth. Just to keep you on your toes, the Greek word for mouth, *stoma* is also used in medical terminology. Put it with *-itis* and you get stomatitis - inflammation of the mouth.

11.24

K14.0 is the code for glossitis.

As you've learned, *gloss-* means the tongue and *-itis* means inflammation. Notice that all K14 codes are for diseases of the tongue. Glance through the indented codes for K14. Did you notice the last two: "Other diseases of tongue" and "Disease of tongue, unspecified"? These two catch-alls, "other" and "unspecified," are common throughout the ICD-10 book.

11.25

Paul sees his doctor about a painful tongue. What code will you use for the doctor's diagnosis, glossodynia?

_____ K14.0   _____ K14.5

_____ K14.4   _____ K14.6

11.26

A common ailment is gastritis, inflammation of the lining of the stomach. What is the code for this condition, if the doctor indicates that it is acute with bleeding?

_____ K29.00   _____ K29.31

_____ K29.01   _____ K29.41

11.27

Lawrence has esophagitis (his esophagus is inflamed). The doctor does not specify any further. Which one of these codes will you choose?

_____ K20   _____ K20.8

_____ K20.0   _____ K20.9

11.28

To complicate matters, Lawrence's esophagus has developed little sacs in the walls, known as diverticulum. Which code is for this condition?

_____ K22.5   _____ K22.4

11.29

Poor Lawrence, he also has dyskinesia, a condition in which the esophagus does not move as it should. What is the code for this condition?

_____ K22.5   _____ K22.4

11.25

K14.6 *Glossodynia* is the best choice.

If you read the handy Greek and Latin boxes at the beginning of this chapter, you'll have no problem with this! As you know, *gloss(o)-* means tongue and the suffix *-dynia* means pain.

11.26

K29.01 is the code for acute gastritis with bleeding.

Of course you know that *gastr-* is Greek for stomach and *-itis* is inflammation.

11.27

K20.9 is the code for esophagitis, unspecified.

11.28

K22.5 is for diverticulum of esophagus, acquired.

Diverticulum are little sacs in the walls of an organ. They bulge out of the organ. They can also be located other places such as the intestines or appendix.

11.29

K22.4 is for dyskinesia of esophagus.

Dyskinesia of esophagus means bad or difficult movement of the esophagus. *Dys-* we learned, means bad, difficult or painful and *-kinesia* comes from the Greek meaning movement.

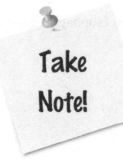

Take Note!

Dyskinesia can affect many organs. For example, K82.8 is for the gallbladder and J98.09 is for the bronchus. (in chapter 10)

11.30

Vaneisha has been diagnosed with duodenal ulcer with hemorrhage.
Dr. Wellbeing's new coder chooses K25.0. Is this the correct code?

_____ Yes   _____ No

11.31

Look at the block of codes for hernia. For the most part, how are the codes in the
hernia block organized?

_____ Alphabetical   _____ By size   _____ By location

11.32

Dr. Wellbeing's first patient this morning was suffering from left sided colitis with
abscess. Which one of these codes will you choose?

_____ K51.011   _____ K51.514   _____ K51.814

11.33

Dr. Wellbeing diagnosed her second patient with eosinophilic gastroenteritis.
There were no additional notes. Which one of these codes will you choose?

_____ K52.9   _____ K52.81   _____ K52.82

11.34

Dr. Wellbeing's third patient this morning has Crohn's disease of the small
intestines. Dr. Wellbeing puts in the notes that there is an intestinal obstruction.
Which of the following codes is correct?

_____ K50.112   _____ K50.00   _____ K50.012

11.30

No, K25.0 is not the correct code for duodenal ulcer with hemorrhage.

The coder missed one key word. K25.0 is *Acute gastric ulcer with hemorrhage.* This patient has a duodenal ulcer. The correct code for this patient is K26.0. Gastric ulcer is K25. Duodenal ulcer is K26.

11.31

The codes in the hernia block are mostly organized by location.

A hernia is a protrusion which can occur in several places in the body, including: the inguinal canal; the femoral canal; the umbilicus or belly button; the abdomen; or the diaphragm. There are other types of hernias listed elsewhere in the ICD-10.

11.32

K51.514 is specifically for left sided colitis with abscess. Notice that you had to look through several colitis codes to get to the most specific one.

Col- is the root word for colon.

11.33

K52.81 is for eosinophilic gastroenteritis.

Enter- means the small intestine. Many times you will see this combined with *gastro-* which means stomach.

11.34

K50.012 is for Crohn's disease of the small intestines with intestinal obstruction.

Look at the indented codes under K50. They are all for Crohn's disease. Notice that the codes indented below K50.0 are for small intestine. The ones indented below K50.1 are for large intestine and the ones indented below K50.8 cover conditions of both small and large intestine at the same time. The codes indented below K50.9 are unspecified.

11.35

Of these four codes, which one is for diverticulitis of the small intestine with perforation and abscess without bleeding?

_____ K57.01   _____ K57.00

_____ K57.20   _____ K57.10

11.36

Which code is for an acute anal fissure?

_____ K60.0   _____ K60.2

_____ K60.1   _____ K60.3

11.37

Which code is for an anal fistula?

_____ K60.0   _____ K60.2

_____ K60.1   _____ K60.3

11.38

Jacob has paralytic ileus, an intestinal obstruction. How will you code it?

_____ K56   _____ K56.1

_____ K56.0   _____ K56.3

11.39

Dr. Wellbeing has a patient with liver failure due to alcohol. The notes say alcoholic hepatic failure with coma. Which code will you use for this condition?

_____ K70.11   _____ K70.40

_____ K70.4   _____ K70.41

11.35

K57.00 is for diverticulitis of the small intestine with perforation and abscess without bleeding.

11.36

K60.0 is the code for an acute anal fissure.

A fissure is a groove, slit or deep furrow.

11.37

K60.3 is the code for an anal fistula.

A fistula is an abnormal passage connecting two body parts.

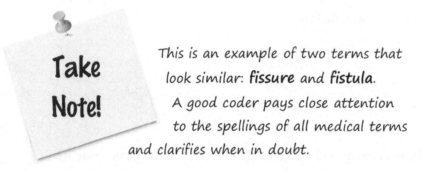

Take Note!

This is an example of two terms that look similar: **fissure** and **fistula**. A good coder pays close attention to the spellings of all medical terms and clarifies when in doubt.

11.38

K56.0 is for paralytic ileus.

Ileus describes a non-mechanical intestinal obstruction, the ability of the intestine to propel matter is affected.

11.39

K70.41 is for alcoholic hepatic failure with coma.

Hepatic pertains to the liver. *Hepa(t)-* is the Greek word for liver and the suffix *-ic* means pertaining to.

11.40

Mr. Brown has chronic persistent hepatitis (inflamed liver) which is not classified elsewhere. Which of these codes applies to this diagnosis?

_____ K73.0   _____ K73.2

_____ K73.1   _____ K73.8

11.41

Ms. Blanca has hepatic sclerosis. Which is the correct code?

_____ K70.2   _____ K74.1

_____ K74.0   _____ K74.2

11.42

Ms. Amarillo was diagnosed with hepatic fibrosis. Which code will you use?

_____ K74.0   _____ K74.2

_____ K74.1   _____ K74.3

11.43

Mr. Green has a colostomy infection. Which of these codes will you use?

_____ K94.00   _____ K94.02

_____ K94.01   _____ K94.09

Take Note!

The suffixes *-iasis* and *-osis* are both Greek words meaning condition or disease. For examples, see K74.0 and K80. But wait. There's also *-pathy* and *-ia*, which mean disease, too.

11.40

<u>K73.0</u> is the code for chronic persistent hepatitis, not elsewhere classified.

Look up hepatitis in the alphabetical index and you will see codes for hepatitis in other chapters. Notice how they are scattered throughout the ICD-10 depending on cause.

 HOT TIP

Like hepatitis, several conditions are scattered throughout the ICD-10. That's one reason it's recommended that you start with the index.

11.41

<u>K74.1</u> is for hepatic sclerosis.

Sclerosis describes a hardening of tissue. Sclerosis comes from the Greek word for "to harden." This is another example of conditions that may not be limited to a single chapter. Sclerosis can occur in many organs or body tissues.

11.42

<u>K74.0</u> is for hepatic fibrosis.

Fibrosis is the abnormal formation of fibrous connective tissue in an organ. In this case, the organ is the liver.

11.43

<u>K94.02</u> is the code for a colostomy infection.

Col- refers to colon and *-stomy* indicates a surgical opening. A colostomy is performed to allow feces to pass from the colon to outside of the body.

11.44

Ms. Haversham is having trouble with her gallbladder. The doctor's diagnosis is acute cholecystitis. Find the correct code?

_____ K80.00   _____ K81.0

_____ K81.1   _____ K81.2

11.45

Ms. Haversham also has cholangitis, which is inflammation of the bile ducts. Which code will you use for this condition?

_____ K83   _____ K83.1

_____ K83.0   _____ K83.9

11.46

Now Ms. Haversham has developed calculus of the gallbladder. The doctor notes that it is with acute cholecystitis without obstruction. Which of these codes will you use?

_____ K80.00   _____ K80.10

_____ K80.01   _____ K80.20

11.47

Complete the code for necrosis of pulp (the center part of the tooth).

K04_____

11.48

One of Dr. Wellbeing's patients has acute recurring sialoadenitis.
Complete the code for this condition.

K1_____

11.44

K81.0 *Acute cholecystitis* is the best choice.

Cholecystitis is inflammation of the gallbladder. *Chole-* comes from the Greek word for bile (which is stored in the gallbladder), *cyst-* means bladder and, of course, *-itis* means inflammation.

 HOT TIP

You're going to love recognizing all these root words. It will make your coding more efficient and more interesting.

11.45

The correct code is K83.0.

Chol- means bile, *ang-* indicates a vessel or duct and *-itis* indicates inflammation.

11.46

K80.00 is for calculus of the gallbladder with acute cholecystitis without obstruction. The clues are: acute, cholecystitis, and without obstruction.

Calculus is another word for stones. K80 *Cholelithiasis* is the condition of having stones in the gallbladder. *Chol-* means bile, *lith-* comes from the Greek word meaning stone, and *-iasis* means condition.

11.47

K04.1 *Necrosis of pulp* is the correct choice.

K04.1 is included in the category for diseases of pulp and periapical tissues.

11.48

The code for *Acute recurring sialoadenitis* is K11.22.

Sialo- = salivary, *aden-* = glands and *-itis* = inflammation. Easy!

11.49

Peter has a femoral hernia, bilateral. There is no obstruction and no gangrene. However, it keeps recurring. Complete the code for this condition.

K_____

11.50

Paula has fibrosis of her pancreas. Complete the code for this condition.

K8_____

11.51

Mary is having a problem with her stomach and esophagus. She has reflux disease and esophagitis. Complete the code for this condition.

K_____

There's a code for THAT??

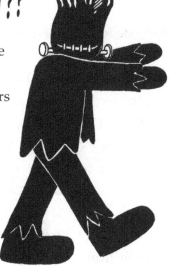

It has been said that beauty is in the eye of the beholder, and ICD-10 apparently agrees. Code R46.1 covers *Bizarre personal appearance.*

11.49

K41.21 is the code for *Bilateral femoral hernia, without obstruction or gangrene, recurrent.*

This might look complicated to code, but it's not, really. Did you locate the block for hernia, and then scan the major hernia codes until you found femoral hernia? The codes for femoral hernia are classified as bilateral (2 sides) and unilateral (1 side). Peter's hernia is bilateral. That means it is either K41.0, K41.1 or K41.2. Looking a little further, find the code worded "without obstruction or gangrene," and then you'll find the code that applies to recurrent.

11.50

The code for fibrosis of the pancreas is K86.89.

The clue K8 allows you to find the pancreas codes quickly. Diseases of the pancreas are codes K85 and K86. You can scan through these codes fairly quickly as there aren't too many. When you get to code K86.89 *Other specified diseases of pancreas*, you can see a list of diseases that are included in that code. Fibrosis of pancreas is included in the list.

11.51

K21.0 is the code for *Gastro-esophageal reflux disease with esophagitis.*

If you look at **Block K20-K31** (Diseases of esophagus, stomach and duodenum), you see that the second entry is K21 for *Gastro-esophageal reflux disease.* This is what is troubling Mary. There are only two codes under K21 – one specifying "with esophagitis" and one specifying "without esophagitis." Mary has esophagitis so choose this code – K21.0.

 HOT TIP

The alphabetical index is a good way to quickly find a code (you then have to follow up by checking the tabular list for notes). You also can use the blocks listed at the beginning of each chapter. For example, you could look up liver in the index, or you can look for the block that contains the liver.

Chapter Quiz (Answers in Appendix A)

Using the Greek and Latin root words in this chapter and Appendix B determine the meaning of the medical terms. Some of the Greek and Latin terms from this chapter are bold.

_____ 11.1	Inflammation of the colon	A.	Dys**kinesia**
_____ 11.2	Little sacs in the walls of an organ	B.	**Diverticul**itis
_____ 11.3	Inflammation of the small intestine	C.	Sialo**lith**iasis
_____ 11.4	Inflammation of mucous membranes	D.	**Proct**itis
_____ 11.5	Difficult movement of an organ	E.	**Gloss**itis
_____ 11.6	Inflammation of the tongue	F.	Fistula
_____ 11.7	Inflammation of the mouth	G.	Mucositis
_____ 11.8	A groove, slit or deep furrow	H.	**Enter**itis
_____ 11.9	Inflammation of the anus	I.	Hypertrophy
_____ 11.10	Calcified stones in a salivary gland	J.	Diverticulum
_____ 11.11	Painful tongue	K.	Peri**odont**itis
_____ 11.12	Inflammation of the esophagus	L.	**Gastr**itis
_____ 11.13	Wasting away of a body part	M.	**Stomat**itis
_____ 11.14	Abnormal passage connecting two body parts	N.	Glosso**dynia**
_____ 11.15	Inflammation of the gums	O.	Sialo**aden**itis
_____ 11.16	Enlargement of a body part	P.	**Col**itis
_____ 11.17	Inflamed little sacs	Q.	**Esophag**itis
_____ 11.18	Inflammation of a salivary gland	R.	Atrophy
_____ 11.19	Inflammation of the lining of the stomach	S.	Fissure
_____ 11.20	Inflammation of tissues surrounding the tooth	T.	**Gingiv**itis

Match the words to the code whose description includes the word.

_____ 11.21 K56.0	A. Fibro**sis**
_____ 11.22 K94.01	B. Hepa**titis**
_____ 11.23 K80.36	C. Chole**lith**iasis
_____ 11.24 K71.10	D. Ileus
_____ 11.25 K40.11	E. Colo**stomy**
_____ 11.26 K52.1	F. **Chol**angitis
_____ 11.27 K80.19	G. Inguinal
_____ 11.28 K13.5	H. Hepa**tic**
_____ 11.29 K80.81	I. Chole**cyst**itis
_____ 11.30 K70.10	J. Gastroenteritis

Match the code to the block title the code is in.

_____ 11.31 K43.2	A. Diseases of oral cavity and salivary glands
_____ 11.32 K35.31	B. Diseases of esophagus, stomach and duodenum
_____ 11.33 K65.1	C. Diseases of appendix
_____ 11.34 K91.1	D. Hernia
_____ 11.35 K29.30	E. Noninfective enteritis and colitis
_____ 11.36 K57.40	F. Other diseases of intestines
_____ 11.37 K74.1	G. Diseases of peritoneum and retroperitoneum
_____ 11.38 K50.813	H. Diseases of liver
_____ 11.39 K80.64	I. Disorders of gallbladder, biliary tract and pancreas
_____ 11.40 K05.1	J. Other diseases of the digestive system

12

Diseases of the Skin and Subcutaneous Tissue

You just completed the digestive system chapter. Are you full? This is a good time to take a break and review some Greek and Latin words in Appendix B before moving on.

Medicine sometimes uses both Greek and Latin roots that mean the same thing. For example, the Greek root word for skin is *derm(a)-* while the Latin root word for skin is *cutis*. The practice of medicine involving the skin is called dermatology, while the skin around the fingernail is called the cuticle.

The first block in this chapter is **L00-L08** (Infections of the skin and subcutaneous tissue). *Sub-* means below (think submarine) and *cutis* means skin; therefore, subcutaneous means below the skin.

Let's look at some of the conditions in the first block. Find L01 *Impetigo*. Impetigo is a contagious bacterial skin infection. Now, browse through the L02 codes and notice that the indented codes are organized by body part:

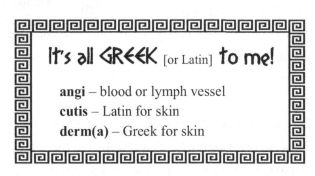

It's all GREEK [or Latin] to me!

angi – blood or lymph vessel
cutis – Latin for skin
derm(a) – Greek for skin

L02.0 (face), L02.1 (neck), L02.2 (trunk), L02.3 (buttock), L02.4 (limb), L02.5 (hand), and L02.6 (foot).

Code L03.0 is *Cellulitis and acute lymphangitis of finger and toe.* We know that both cellulitis and lymphangitis are inflammations because they end in *-itis*. Notice that the codes indented beneath L03 are organized by body part, similar to, but differently than the codes indented under L02.

The second block in this chapter is **L10–L14** (Bullous disorders). What's a bullous disorder? *Bullous* comes from the Latin for bubble. In medical terminology, it means a blister filled with fluid.

You already know how to break down dermatitis. *Derma-* = skin and *-itis* = inflammation, so, dermatitis is inflammation of the skin. **Block L20-L30** covers dermatitis and eczema. Find this block in your ICD-10 and read the beginning note. It tells you that in this block dermatitis and eczema will mean the same thing.

Let's look at the intimidating medical term "papulosquamous." It is made of two parts: the Latin word *papulo-* meaning red elevated areas on the skin called papules (pimples) and *-squamous* from the Latin for scale-like. So, papulosquamous means having characteristics of both papules (pimples) and scales. **L40-L45** is a block for Papulosquamous disorders.

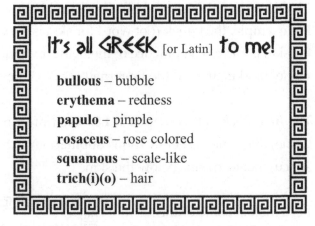

It's all GREEK [or Latin] to me!

bullous – bubble
erythema – redness
papulo – pimple
rosaceus – rose colored
squamous – scale-like
trich(i)(o) – hair

The block following papulosquamous disorders is **L49-L54** (Urticaria and erythema). Urticaria is a type of skin rash. *Erythema* comes from the Greek word meaning redness and refers to redness of the skin.

Check out **Block L55-L59** (Radiation-related disorders of the skin and subcutaneous tissue). You might find it surprising that sunburn is not coded as a burn in Chapter 19. It is considered a radiation related disorder! See code L55.

Block L60-L75 reveals another fascinating factoid. According to ICD-10, nails, hair, acne, pimples, hair follicles and even sweat glands are all considered skin appendages.

What happens when a condition does not fit into any block? Many chapters of the ICD-10 include a block for conditions that do not fit. ICD-10 often resolves this at the end of the chapter. For example, the last block in this chapter is **L80-L99** (Other disorders of the skin and subcutaneous tissue). The first code, L80 *Vitiligo* is loss of skin pigmentation. Code L81 is *Other disorders of pigmentation*.

Find code L89 *Pressure ulcer*. There are many codes indented beneath L89, all organized by body part. Have you noticed that organizing by body part is a common scheme used in the ICD-10?

Referring to your ICD-10 book and your Greek and Latin root words in Appendix B, see how much you can deduce in the following exercises:

12.1
What does subcutaneous mean?

_____ Above the skin   _____ On the skin
_____ Below the skin   _____ Tissue other than skin

12.2
What does the Greek root word *derm(a)-* refer to?

_____ Skin   _____ Above the skin
_____ Tissue other than skin _____ Below the skin

12.3
What's the first letter of all codes for diseases of the skin and subcutaneous tissue?

_____

12.4
Find code L01 in your ICD-10 book. This code is for what condition?

_____ Impetigo   _____ Cellulitis   _____ Lymphangitis   _____ Lymphadenitis

12.1

Subcutaneous means <u>below the skin</u>.

Sub- means below and *-cutis*
means skin. Therefore, sub +
cutaneous means below the
skin.

12.2

Derm(a)- is a word part that
means <u>skin</u>.

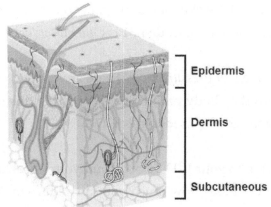

Many medical words,
diagnoses and procedures begin with *derm(a)-*.

12.3

All codes for the skin and subcutaneous tissue section begin with the letter <u>L</u>.

12.4

<u>*Impetigo*</u> is code L01 in the ICD-10.

QUICK QUIZ *Answers in Appendix A*	
_____ 12.1 Pain	*A.* -stomy
_____ 12.2 Condition	*B.* -dynia
_____ 12.3 Pertaining to	*C.* -ic
_____ 12.4 Surgical opening	*D.* -iasis

12.5

Moe has a condition that was coded L03.011. What condition did his doctor diagnose?

_____ Impetigo   _____ Cellulitis   _____ Lymphangitis   _____ Lymphadenitis

12.6

Larry has a condition listed as L03.022. Which condition is this code for?

_____ Impetigo   _____ Cellulitis   _____ Lymphangitis   _____ Lymphadenitis

12.7

Curly's claim was coded L04.0. What does the doctor call this condition?

_____ Impetigo   _____ Cellulitis   _____ Lymphangitis   _____ Lymphadenitis

12.8

The second block in the skin and subcutaneous tissue chapter covers bullous disorders. Which of the following diagnosis codes can be found in this block?

_____ L10   _____ L11
_____ L12   _____ L13
_____ L14   _____ All of these

12.9

Find the block in your ICD-10 book for papulosquamous disorders. Which of the following is an example of a papulosquamous disorder?

_____ Psoriasis   _____ Parapsoriasis
_____ Lichen planus   _____ Lichen striatus
_____ All of these

12.5

L03.011 is for _Cellulitis of right finger_.

Cellulitis is a bacterial infection spreading just below the skin surface. Look at the codes indented beneath L03 and notice how many there are for cellulitis.

12.6

L03.022 is for _Acute lymphangitis of left finger_.

Lymphangitis is infection and inflammation of the lymphatic channels. Let's break this big word down. **_Lymph-_** refers to the lymphatic system. **_Angi-_** means a blood or lymph vessel and **_-itis_**, as you know, means inflammation. Notice how the codes in L03 are structured. They are organized by body part, first for cellulitis and then for lymphangitis.

12.7

L04.0 is _Acute lymphadenitis_. L04.01 covers face, head and neck.

Lymphadenitis is inflammation of a lymph node. **_Lymph-_** refers to the lymphatic system. **_Adeno-_** means gland. **_-itis_** means inflammation. Easy!

12.8

The correct answer is <u>all of these</u>.

A bullous disorder is a large blister filled with fluid. There are five sub-codes for bullous disorders. They are listed as codes L10 - L14.

12.9

<u>All of these</u> are examples of papulosquamous disorders.

Psoriasis is L40, _Parapsoriasis_ is L41, _Lichen planus_ is L43 and _Lichen striatus_ is L44.2.

12.10

May goes to her doctor with a skin rash characterized by red bumps. Her diagnosis is allergic urticaria. Which code best covers this condition?

_____ L50.0   _____ L51.8   _____ L55.0   _____ L57.0

12.11

Scarlett's doctor diagnosed her condition as a type of erythema. Which of these codes will you use?

_____ L50.0   _____ L51.8   _____ L55.0   _____ L57.0

12.12

What do you code the diagnosis of follicular disorder, unspecified?

_____ L64.8   _____ L71.9   _____ L73.9   _____ L68.9

12.13

Which code is for rosacea due to an unspecified cause?

_____ L71.0   _____ L71.1   _____ L71.8   _____ L71.9

12.14

Bill is losing his hair. The diagnosis is drug induced androgenic alopecia. Which of these codes will you use?

_____ L63.8   _____ L64.0
_____ L64.8   _____ L64.9

There's a code for THAT??

If the patient has spent too much time with his winged-friends, he may be suffering from J67.2 *Bird fancier's lung*.

12.10

Code <u>L50.0</u> is for allergic urticaria.

Look up L50 in your ICD-10 and notice there are several types of urticaria.

12.11

The correct code is <u>L51.8</u>.

Erythema, redness of the skin caused by superficial capillaries, comes from the Greek word meaning red. Blushing is a non-medical example of erythema.

12.12

<u>L73.9</u> is the correct code.

Follicular pertains to a small sac or cavity such as one from which a hair develops. Follicular disorders are covered by codes L72 and L73.

12.13

<u>L71.9</u> *Rosacea, unspecified* is the correct code.

Rosacea is a chronic skin disorder of the face characterized by redness and pimples. Rosacea is derived from the Latin word for rosy.

12.14

<u>L64.0</u> *Drug induced androgenic alopecia* is the correct code.

Alopecia is hair loss. The most common form of alopecia is male pattern baldness.

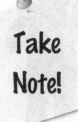

Take Note!

*The block **L60-L75** (Disorders of skin appendages) is very broad, and includes codes for conditions relating to hair loss, hair color, nails, acne, rosacea, follicle disorders and sweat gland disorders.*

12.15

Stuart has hypertrichosis, an abnormal amount of hair growth over his body but there are no specifics on the chart. Which of these codes apply in this situation?

_____ L68.1   _____ L68.2   _____ L68.9   _____ L73.9

12.16

Raj has been diagnosed with epidermal thickening with no other specifics on the chart. How should you code it?

_____ L85   _____ L85.9
_____ L85.8   _____ L86

12.17

Leonard has been bedridden for months, the friction on his skin has resulted in a stage 1 pressure ulcer of his upper right back. Which one of these codes applies to this situation?

_____ L89.101   _____ L89.121
_____ L89.111   _____ L89.131

12.18

Penny sees her dermatologist for an inflamed, noncancerous skin growth on her back known as a seborrheic keratosis. Which one of these codes will you use?

_____ L82   _____ L82.0
_____ L82.1   _____ L83

12.19

Amy consults her dermatologist for a skin pigment condition which the doctor diagnosed as vitiligo. What is the code for this condition?

_____ L80   _____ L81.2
_____ L81   _____ L81.6

12.15

L68.9 *Hypertrichosis, unspecified* is the best choice.

Hyper- means excess. *Trich-* means hair. *-osis* means condition.

12.16

L85.9 *Epidermal thickening, unspecified* is the best choice.

Epidermal refers to the outermost layer of skin. *Epi-* means upon or over and *-dermal* refers to the skin.

12.17

L89.111 is the code for a stage 1 pressure ulcer of the upper right back.

Because there are many locations where patients can have pressure ulcers, there are many pressure ulcer codes under L89 in the ICD-10.

 HOT TIP

Pressure ulcers are easier to code once you realize they're organized by body part!

12.18

L82.0 is the code for inflamed seborrheic keratosis.

Seborrheic keratoses are noncancerous skin growths. They increase as people age.

12.19

L80 is the code for vitiligo.

Vitiligo is the condition in which parts of the skin become depigmented. It occurs when skin pigment cells die or do not function properly.

12.20

Can a neoplasm (C00-D49) be used on the same claim as a code from the chapter entitled Diseases of the Skin and Subcutaneous Tissue?

_____ Yes   _____ No

12.21

You see a claim for L01.01 *Non-bullous impetigo.* Also coded on the claim is L40.1 *Impetigo herpatiformis.* Can these two codes be used on the same claim?

_____ Yes   _____ No

12.22

The patient has a pressure ulcer on the right upper back. Gangrene is involved. Which of the following is the correct way to code this?

_____ I96 and then L89.114   _____ L89.114 and then I96

12.23

You see a claim with L02.31 *Cutaneous abscess of buttock* listed first and L05.01 *Pilonidal cyst with abscess* listed second. Is this the correct way to code this?

_____ Yes, cutaneous abscess of buttock should be coded first
_____ No, pilonidal cyst with abscess should be coded first
_____ No, these codes should not be used together

12.24

What is the code for pemphigus vegetans? Hint: if you don't have a clear idea where to look for a code, go to the alphabetical index.

_____

12.20

<u>Yes</u>, neoplasms and any code from the Diseases of the Skin and Subcutaneous Tissue chapter can be listed together.

How do you know? There is an **Excludes2** note at the beginning of the Diseases of the Skin and Subcutaneous Tissue chapter. Always read the notes! This one advises that neoplasms are not part of the conditions in this chapter, so both conditions may be coded.

12.21

<u>No</u>, L01.01 and L40.1 cannot be coded together.

The **Excludes1** note after L01 *Impetigo* excludes *Impetigo herpatiformis* (L40.1). So the two codes cannot be used at the same time.

12.22

The correct order to code these is <u>I96 and then L89.114</u>.

Look at the notes after code L89. The **"Code first"** note says "Code first any associated gangrene (I96)." Therefore, the proper coding is I96 first and then L89.114.

12.23

The correct answer is <u>no, these codes should not be used together</u>.

Why not? Look at the notes after code L02.3. The **Excludes1** note lists *Pilonidal cyst with abscess* (L05.01). Therefore, these two codes should not be used together.

12.24

The code for *Pemphigus vegetans* is <u>L10.1</u>.

Did you start at the alphabetical index? If so, you looked up pemphigus and saw several entries. You scanned the entries and found vegetans. Good job! Remember, after you find the code, go to the chapter and check for notes.

For these practice questions use the alphabetical index to look up these codes and then verify the code in the tabular list.

12.25

Leroy's doctor diagnosed him with acrodermatitis continua. What is the code for this condition?

_____

12.26

Mr. Blaze has pale red bumps on his skin that itch. The doctor calls this condition allergic urticaria (commonly known as hives). What is the code for allergic urticaria?

_____

12.27

Ms. Rivers has a condition involving excessive sweating of her face. The doctor diagnosed this condition as primary focal hyperhidrosis of the face. What is the code for this condition?

_____

12.28

Mr. Lakes has a skin condition his doctor diagnosed as impetigo that is non-bullous. What is the code for this condition?

_____

QUICK QUIZ *Answers in Appendix A*		
_____ 12.5 Certain Infectious and Parasitic Diseases	*A.*	C18.8
_____ 12.6 Neoplasms	*B.*	E05.8
_____ 12.7 Diseases of the Blood and Blood-forming Organs	*C.*	A87.1
_____ 12.8 Endocrine, Nutritional, and Metabolic Diseases	*D.*	D57.211

12.25

The code for *Acrodermatitis continua* is <u>L40.2.</u>

When searching the index, you'll see several entries under acrodermatitis. Look for continua and you'll find code L40.2. Once you find it in the alphabetical index, always look up the code in the tabular list so you can check for notes.

12.26

The code for *Allergic urticaria* is <u>L50.0.</u>

Look up urticaria or allergic in the alphabetical index. Find the exact diagnosis you are looking for and you will see the code – L50.0.

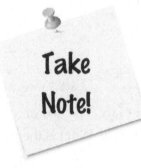

Take Note!

Remember: don't rely totally on the alphabetical index! There may be notes in the tabular list that will affect your code.

12.27

The code for *Primary focal hyperhidrosis of the face* is <u>L74.511</u>.

Find the key medical term to look up in the index; in this case, it's hyperhidrosis. Then look for focal, and then primary, and then face and you will find the code, L74.511. And then find the code in the tabular list and check for notes.

12.28

The code for *Non-bullous impetigo* is <u>L01.01</u>.

If you look up non-bullous in the index, you won't find it. It is best practice to look up the condition in the index (in this case, impetigo) and then read the descriptors that make the condition unique. Notice the list of types of impetigo, now find nonbullous and go to the chapter and check for notes.

12.29

Samuel has lymphadenitis. It is affecting the upper part of his right arm near the shoulder and is acute. What is the code for this condition?

_____

12.30

Eva tried a new brand of cosmetics and got a bad case of allergic contact dermatitis. What is the code for this condition?

_____

12.31

A bedridden patient in a nursing home has a non-pressure ulcer of her left ankle. This is a chronic condition for this patient. There's no necrosis but the fat layer is exposed. What is the code for this condition?

_____

12.32

Ursula had a dermatological surgical procedure performed yesterday. Today she's having a problem with postprocedural hemorrhage of the skin and subcutaneous tissue. What is the correct code for this?

_____

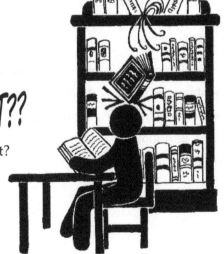

There's a code for THAT??

Nice, quiet libraries are pretty safe, right? Apparently not always. ICD-10's code Y92.241 covers occurrences at libraries.

12.29

The code for *Acute lymphadenitis of upper limb* is <u>L04.2</u>.

First, look up the condition lymphadenitis in the alphabetical index. Find acute, and then look for limb and upper and you will find the code. Remember to look up the code in the tabular list and check for notes. In this case, there are both an **Includes** note and an **Excludes1** note associated with L04.

12.30

The code for *Allergic contact dermatitis due to cosmetics* is <u>L23.2</u>.

Under dermatitis in the index, look up contact. Under contact, look for allergic, and then "due to cosmetics." Once you have the code, check for notes. You'll find **Excludes1** and **Excludes2** notes with L23.

12.31

The code for *Non-pressure chronic ulcer of left ankle with fat layer exposed* is <u>L97.322</u>.

In the index, look up ulcer. The ankle is part of the lower limb, so you need to find lower limb and then ankle. This is the left ankle, so find left, and then find "with exposed fat layer." Once you have the code, you know what to do: look up the code in the tabular list and check for notes.

12.32

The code for *Postprocedural hemorrhage of skin and subcutaneous tissue following a dermatologic procedure* is <u>L76.21</u>.

The block covering intraoperative and postprocedural complications of skin and subcutaneous tissue is **(L76)**. Ursula's condition falls into this block as it was a complication following a procedure. It is a rather small block so you can browse it quickly and look for postprocedural hemorrhage and then look for "following a dermatologic procedure."

Chapter Quiz (Answers in Appendix A)

Using your knowledge of Greek and Latin roots, match the definition to the term found in this chapter. Some of the Greek and Latin terms from this chapter are bold.

_____ 12.1	Below the skin	A. Sub**cutaneous**
_____ 12.2	Inflammation of the lymphatic channels	B. Epi**derm**al
_____ 12.3	Outermost layer of skin	C. Lymph**angi**tis
_____ 12.4	Psoriasis is an example of this	D. Hyper**trich**osis
_____ 12.5	Abnormal amount of hair growth	E. Papulo**squamous** disorder

Match the words to the code whose description includes the word(s).

_____ 12.6	L01.02	A.	Follicular
_____ 12.7	L50.3	B.	Dermatitis
_____ 12.8	L03.019	C.	Lymphadenitis
_____ 12.9	L72.9	D.	Rosacea
_____ 12.10	L63.1	E.	Bullous
_____ 12.11	L30.4	F.	Urticaria
_____ 12.12	L12.0	G.	Erythema
_____ 12.13	L71.8	H.	Pressure ulcer
_____ 12.14	L04.2	I.	Impetigo
_____ 12.15	L89.002	J.	Alopecia
_____ 12.16	L21.1	K.	Vitiligo
_____ 12.17	L82.1	L.	Cellulitis
_____ 12.18	L80	M.	Seborrheic keratosis

Use the alphabetical index to find the code for each description.

_____ 12.19 Acquired epidermolysis bullosa, unspecified

_____ 12.20 Small plaque parapsoriasis

_____ 12.21 Acute radiodermatitis

_____ 12.22 Pressure ulcer of left heel, stage 4

_____ 12.23 Furuncle of head [any part, except face]

_____ 12.24 Irritant contact dermatitis due to solvents

_____ 12.25 Other rosacea

_____ 12.26 Allergic urticaria

_____ 12.27 Folliculitis ulerythematosa reticulata

Indicate all appropriate notes for each code.

12.28 L43.2 _____ _____ _____   A. **Includes**

12.29 L10.81 _____ _____   B. **Excludes1**

12.30 L76.81 _____ _____   C. **Excludes2**

12.31 L57.1 _____ _____   D. **"Use additional code"**

12.32 L01.01 _____ _____ _____   E. **"Code first"**

12.33 L82.0 _____ _____

12.34 L60.1 _____ _____

12.35 L04.2 _____ _____ _____ _____

12.36 L49.1 _____ _____ _____

12.37 L93.0 _____ _____ _____

12.38 L23.3 _____ _____ _____

13

Diseases of the Musculoskeletal System and Connective Tissue

This chapter is about conditions of the muscles, joints and bones. For example, arthritis, bursitis and gout. Before we get started, please read the note at the beginning of Chapter 13 in the ICD-10-CM. It tells you that if there is an external cause for the condition (such as an accident), you should follow the code from this chapter with an external cause code from Chapter 20.

As we go through this chapter, we'll look at some new words related to diseases of the musculoskeletal system and connective tissue. Breaking down the word arthropathy for example, you start with *arthro-*, which comes from a Greek word meaning joint. The suffix *–pathy* indicates a disease. Therefore, arthropathy indicates a disease of the joint.

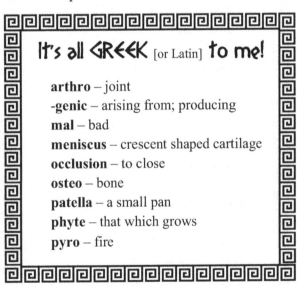

It's all GREEK [or Latin] to me!

arthro – joint
-genic – arising from; producing
mal – bad
meniscus – crescent shaped cartilage
occlusion – to close
osteo – bone
patella – a small pan
phyte – that which grows
pyro – fire

The first block in this chapter, **M00-M02**, covers infectious arthropathies. If you put *poly-* in front of arthropathies, what does the new word mean? *Poly-* you recall means many, so polyarthropathies means that more than one joint is involved. The second block in this chapter, **M05-M14**, covers inflammatory arthropathies.

Osteoarthritis is a type of arthritis. *Osteo-*, from a Greek word meaning bone, indicates that the arthritis is characterized by involvement of the bone and the joint. You can find it in **Block M15-M19.** Look up the first code in this block: M15 *Polyosteoarthritis.* There's that prefix *poly-* again. It indicates that osteoarthritis exists in many areas.

Block M26-M27 covers the jaws and teeth. Be vigilant on this one! There are only two categories in this block, M26 and M27, but it has many indented codes.

In the next block, systemic connective tissue disorders (**M30-M36**) the conditions involve connective tissue throughout the body. For example, M32 *Systemic lupus erythematosus (SLE)* is not localized to one area of the body.

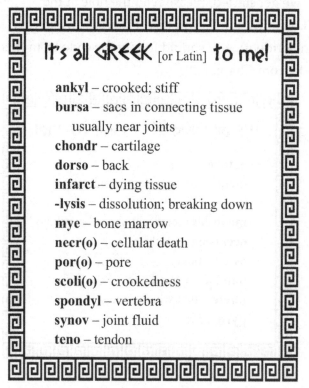

It's all GREEK [or Latin] **to me!**

ankyl – crooked; stiff
bursa – sacs in connecting tissue
    usually near joints
chondr – cartilage
dorso – back
infarct – dying tissue
-lysis – dissolution; breaking down
mye – bone marrow
necr(o) – cellular death
por(o) – pore
scoli(o) – crookedness
spondyl – vertebra
synov – joint fluid
teno – tendon

The term *dorso-* comes from a Latin word meaning back. The suffix *-pathy*, as you know, means disorder or disease. The Greek word *spondyl-* means vertebra. So, dorsopathy means a disorder or disease of the back and spondylopathy is a condition of the vertebra. The three blocks, **M40-M43** (Deforming dorsopathies), **M45-M49** (Spondylopathies) and **M50-M54** (Other dorsopathies) cover diagnoses related to the back and spine.

Take a look at **Block M65-M67** (Disorders of synovium and tendon). *Synov-* is the root Latin word for the synovial membrane. The term *teno-* is a Greek word for tendon. A condition that occurs many times in this block is tenosynovitis – inflammation of the tendon and synovial membrane.

This block is followed by **M70-M79** (Other soft tissue disorders). You will notice that the most common diagnosis is bursitis, inflammation of the bursa.

Block M80-M85 covers disorders of bone density and structure. One of the common diagnoses you will see here is osteoporosis. It's a condition in which the bones are losing density and becoming more breakable. *Osteo-* means bone, and *-porosis* refers to pore.

The next block, **M86-M90**, covers other osteopathies. Osteopathies means diseases of the bone.

Chondropathies are diseases of the cartilage. For example, in **Block M91-M94** (Chondropathies) the first code is M91 *Juvenile osteochondrosis of hip and pelvis*. When you break down the word osteochondrosis, you get *osteo-* (bone), *chondr-* (cartilage) and *-osis* (condition).

Here are some practice exercises using the M codes.

13.1
In the first block you'll see infectious arthropathies. Based on the root words, what does arthropathy mean?

_____ Disease of the muscle   _____ Disease of the connective tissue
_____ Disease of the joint   _____ Disease of the bone

13.2
You know that *pyro-* means fire and *-genic* means producing. What does pyrogenic in code M00 *Pyrogenic arthritis* mean?

_____ Producing a fever   _____ Not able to move
_____ Coming from the joint   _____ Painful when moved

13.3
Polyarthropathies is a long word, but with the Greek and Latin roots it breaks down this way: poly-arthro-pathies. What does polyarthropathies mean?

_____ Disease involving one joint
_____ Disease involving more than one joint
_____ Disease involving both the joint and bone

13.1

Arthropathy means <u>disease of the joint</u>.

Arthro- is from the Greek word for joint. *-pathy* means disease.

13.2

Pyrogenic means <u>producing a fever</u>.

Pyro means fire in Greek, and *-genic* means producing. If you've ever had a fever, you know that it feels like you're on fire!

13.3

Polyarthropathies are <u>diseases involving more than one joint</u>.

Poly- means many. *Arthro-* is from the Greek word for joint. *-pathy* means disease.

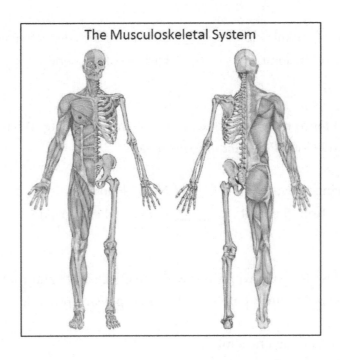

The Musculoskeletal System

13.4

Browse through the block covering inflammatory polyarthropathies (**M05-M14**). Which of the following has the most indented codes?

_____ M05 *Rheumatoid arthritis with*   _____ M06 *Other rheumatoid*
      rheumatoid factor   *arthritis*

_____ M07 *Enteropathic arthropathies*   _____ M08 *Juvenile arthritis*

13.5

What does *osteo-* mean?

_____ Joint   _____ Bone

_____ Muscle   _____ Connective tissue

13.6

Patella is a new word in this chapter. It comes from the Latin word for a small pan, in non-medical terms the kneecap. Choose the code involving the patella.

_____ M02.811   _____ M22.02

_____ M31.3   _____ M80.041

13.7

Code M23 involves the meniscus, a crescent shaped cartilage found in certain joints. Which joint in this chapter involves the meniscus?

_____ Hip   _____ Knee

_____ Ankle   _____ Elbow

13.8

Mr. Habblegaber has been diagnosed with osteomyelitis, inflammation of the bone and bone marrow of vertebra in the thoracic region. Which one of these codes is most appropriate?

_____ M42.02   _____ M46.24

_____ M46.85   _____ M47.9

13.4

M05 *Rheumatoid arthritis with rheumatoid factor* has more indented codes than the others.

There are many codes for arthritis. Of the four categories listed, M05 *Rheumatoid arthritis with rheumatoid factor* has the most.

13.5

Osteo- means bone.

Osteoarthritis is the most common form of arthritis. It is characterized by destruction of the joint.

13.6

Code M22.02 involves the patella.

The patella is the kneecap.

13.7

The knee has several codes involving meniscus.

The word meniscus comes from the Greek word for crescent.

13.8

M46.24 *Osteomyelitis of vertebra, thoracic region* is the correct code.

Osteo- = bone; *mye--* = bone marrow and *-itis* = inflammation.

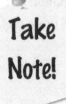 **Take Note!**

Don't confuse *mye* (bone marrow) with *myel* (spine) or *myo* (muscle). Many Greek and Latin word parts look alike and/or sound alike.

13.9

Ms. Lincoln has abnormal rigidity and immobility of the joint in her right wrist, known as ankylosis. Which is the best code for this condition?

_____ M24.63   _____ M24.632

_____ M24.631   _____ M24.671

13.10

Mr. Adams has a condition involving bleeding into the joints. The doctor has diagnosed it as hemarthrosis of the left hand. How will you code it?

_____ M25.00   _____ M25.041

_____ M25.04   _____ M25.042

13.11

Ms. Washington has fluid escaping into an elbow joint. The doctor's notes say "effusion, right elbow." Which of these is the correct code for this condition?

_____ M25.042   _____ M25.422

_____ M25.421   _____ M25.471

13.12

Mr. Jefferson has back problems. His doctor indicated a diagnosis of "spondylolysis, lumbar region." Which one of these codes should you use?

_____ M43.07   _____ M43.16

_____ M43.06   _____ M43.17

13.13

Ms. Franklin's teeth do not align when her jaws close. You are instructed to code it as malocclusion, Angle's class II. Find the proper code.

_____ M26.211   _____ M26.212

_____ M26.213   _____ M26.219

13.9

<u>M24.631</u> is the best choice.

Ankylosis is the condition of having stiff joints. *Ankyl-* comes from the Greek word for crooked or stiff, and *-osis* means condition. Notice that the indented codes under M24.6 are organized by location in the body.

13.10

<u>M25.042</u> *Hemarthrosis, left hand* is the best choice.

Hemarthrosis is the condition of bleeding into a joint. *Hem-* means blood. *Arthr-* means joint. *-osis* means condition. Look at code M25.0 and notice the codes indented beneath it are organized by location in the body.

13.11

<u>M25.421</u> is the code for effusion, right elbow.

Effusion means fluid escaping into a body part. The fluid can be escaping into the pleural cavity or other body part. In this case it is flowing into a joint.

13.12

<u>M43.06</u> is the code for spondylolysis, lumbar region.

Spondyl- means vertebra. *-lysis* means dissolution or breaking down.

13.13

<u>M26.212</u> is for malocclusion, Angle's class II.

Mal- comes from Greek and means bad. Occlusion is the manner in which the teeth meet when they close. Malocclusion means the teeth do not align when the person's jaws close. The block of codes **M26-M27** is for Dentofacial anomalies [including malocclusion] and other disorders of jaw.

13.14

Mr. Hancock has a curved spine diagnosed as neuromuscular scoliosis. The doctor's notes specifies it as the lumbar region. Which code applies?

_____ M41.26   _____ M41.47

_____ M41.46   _____ M41.86

13.15

Which code is for polyarteritis nodosa, a condition in which many arteries are inflamed?

_____ M30   _____ M30.0

_____ M30.1   _____ M30.2

13.16

Mr. Markham has an osteophyte, which is a bone spur in his left shoulder. Which one of these codes will you use?

_____ M25.721   _____ M25.711

_____ M25.722   _____ M25.712

13.17

Mr. Grant has inflammatory spondylopathies of the thoracolumbar region. Which one of these codes is appropriate for the claim?

_____ M46.27   _____ M46.80

_____ M46.85   _____ M46.84

13.18

Hector, age 7, has a condition called spinal osteochondrosis. The doctor indicates that it involves the cervical region. Which one of these codes will you use?

_____ M46.24   _____ M42.02

_____ M46.85   _____ M47.9

13.14

<u>M41.26</u> is the code for neuromuscular scoliosis, lumbar region.

Scoliosis comes from the Greek word for crookedness. It is a condition in which the spine curves, sometimes forming an S shape. Look at the indented codes under M41 for scoliosis codes and notice that at the most detailed level they are divided by spinal region.

13.15

<u>M30.0</u> is the code for polyarteritis nodosa.

Poly- = many; *arter-* = artery and *-itis* = inflammation.

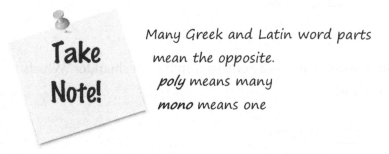

Take Note!

Many Greek and Latin word parts mean the opposite.
poly means many
mono means one

13.16

<u>M25.712</u> is the code for osteophyte, left shoulder.

Osteo- means bone. *-phyte* comes from a Greek word for "that which grows."

13.17

<u>M46.85</u> is the best choice.

Spondyl- = vertebra and *-pathies* = diseases or conditions. You'll find these codes in **Block M45-M49**.

13.18

<u>M42.02</u> is the code for juvenile osteochondrosis of spine, cervical region.

The root words are *osteo-* = bone; *-chondr-* = cartilage and *-osis* = condition.

13.19

Which code is for the breaking down of a vertebral structure in the lumbar region?

_____ M48.06   _____ M47.895

_____ M48.07   _____ M47.896

Moving on to the soft tissue disorders section, let's do some research in codes M60-M79.

13.20

The patient has been diagnosed with nontraumatic ischemic infarction of the right hand. What is the code?

_____ M62.211   _____ M62.231

_____ M62.221   _____ M62.241

13.21

Ms. White has myositis, an inflammation of her left thigh muscle. Which one of these codes is most appropriate?

_____ M60.022   _____ M60.042

_____ M60.032   _____ M60.052

13.22

Professor Plum has been diagnosed with olecranon bursitis of his left elbow. Which one of these codes will you choose?

_____ M70.20   _____ M70.22

_____ M70.21   _____ M70.32

13.23

Mrs. Peacock visits her doctor because she has pain in her wrist. The doctor diagnosed synovitis, but he didn't specify which wrist. Which code is best?

_____ M65.131   _____ M65.139

_____ M65.132   _____ M65.149

13.19

M47.896 is the code for "other spondylosis, lumbar region."

Spondylosis is the breaking down of a vertebral structure. *Spondyl-* = vertebra and *-lysis* = dissolution. As you become accustomed to the root words, you'll find these complicated medical terms easy to recognize.

13.20

M62.241 is the code for a nontraumatic ischemic infarction of a muscle in the right hand.

Isch- is from the Greek meaning restriction; *hemic-* means blood. An *infarct* is an area of tissue in a body that is dying. Notice that these codes, like many codes in this chapter, are organized by body part: shoulder, upper arm, forearm, hand, thigh, leg, lower leg, ankle and foot.

13.21

M60.052 is the best choice. Myositis is a term for inflammation of the muscle.

Myo- is Greek for muscle; *-itis* = inflammation. Notice that there are many indented codes under M60, so ICD-10 requires you to be very specific!

13.22

M70.22 is the best choice. Bursitis is the inflammation of the bursa.

Bursa are sacs in connecting tissue usually near joints. Check out all the various codes for bursitis. It is common for ICD-10 to be organized as: right, left and unspecified for some body parts.

13.23

M65.139 is the best choice.

Synov- refers to the synovial membrane, which lines the capsule of joints. When this membrane becomes inflamed, it is called synovitis.

13.24

Mrs. Wiggins, age 75, had a recent fracture of her left forearm. The chart includes osteoporosis as a factor. Which one of these codes will you use?

_____ M80.022   _____ M80.032

_____ M80.031   _____ M80.039

13.25

Stan's bone cells are dying due to an interruption of the blood supply. His doctor diagnosed idiopathic aseptic osteonecrosis of the left humerus. Choose the best code for this condition.

_____ M87.011   _____ M87.019

_____ M87.012   _____ M87.022

13.26

According to Mary Lou's chart, she has osteomalacia due to malnutrition. Which one of the following codes will you use?

_____ M83.2   _____ M83.5

_____ M83.3   _____ M83.8

13.27

Carl has a type of osteitis of the left shoulder known as osteitis deformans. Which one of the following codes will you use for this condition?

_____ M80.012   _____ M85.311

_____ M80.812   _____ M88.812

13.28

You see a claim for a young boy that has been coded with both M08.1 _Juvenile ankylosing spondylitis_ and M45.2 _Ankylosing spondylitis of cervical region_. Is this the correct way to code this?

_____ Yes, M45.2 further clarifies the region affected
_____ No, these two codes should not be used together
_____ Maybe, I'm not sure

13.24

M80.032 is the correct choice.

Osteoporosis occurs when the bones lose density and become more porous. *Osteo-* means bone and *-porosis* is from the Greek meaning porous.

13.25

M87.022 is the correct answer.

Osteo- means bone and *-necrosis* means cellular death (Not your phone, cells of the body). Take a look at code M87 and check out the indented codes for osteonecrosis. They are organized both by cause of necrosis and by location.

13.26

The answer is M83.3 *Adult osteomalacia due to malnutrition.*

Osteomalacia is softening of the bones. *Osteo-* means bone and *-malacia* indicates softening. You can find other codes for osteomalacia under M83.

13.27

M88.812 is the best choice.

Osteitis is inflammation of the bone. You already know both word parts: *Oste-* = bone; *-itis* = inflammation. Look up osteitis in the index. Notice the many different types of osteitis listed.

13.28

No, these two codes (M08.1 and M45.2) should not be used together.

When you look up code M45 *Ankylosing spondylitis*, you'll see an important **Excludes1** note that says you cannot use any of the M45 codes with M08.1. The claim should be coded with only M08.1. Always check those notes!

13.29

A 55-year old woman has a ganglion of her right knee. She also has a synovial cyst of popliteal space of her right knee. Which is the correct way to code her claim?

_____ M67.461 only   _____ M71.21 only   _____ M67.461 and M71.21

13.30

A 62-year old man has staphylococcal arthritis of the left hip. The cause is a methicillin susceptible Staphylococcus aureus infection. The claim has both codes M00.052 and B95.61. Is this coded correctly?

_____ Yes, both can be used on the same claim
_____ No, there is an **Excludes1** note associated with M00.052

13.31

A 47-year old man has rheumatoid arthritis of his right shoulder with involvement of other organs. The claim is coded M05.611 and I00. Can these two codes be used together?

_____ Yes, it is ok to code these together
_____ No, there is an **Excludes1** note

13.32

Mr. Bonono has idiopathic gout of his left elbow. It is a chronic condition. He has a tophus on the elbow. What will the doctor's coder use for his diagnosis?
(HINT: pay special attention to the note about 7th characters under M1A. Use of any codes that begin with M1A require using a 7th character. Instructions for the 7th character are provided under the M1A code. This is a great time to review the "Anatomy of a code" section of the Basic Concepts chapter in this book, pages 3-6.)

M1A._____

13.29

The correct way to code this case is <u>M67.461 and M71.21</u>.

Look up code M67.461 *Ganglion, right knee*. Now, search back to M67.4 *Ganglion* and look for any notes that would apply to code M67.461. There is an **Excludes1** note and an **Excludes2** note associated with M67.4. The **Excludes1** note does not affect this claim, but the **Excludes2** note does. It lists M71.2, which means that both conditions may be coded together.

13.30

<u>Yes, both (M00.052 and B95.61) can used on the same claim</u>.

Look at the note under code M00.0. It says "Use additional code (B95.61-B95.8) to identify bacterial agent." Not only can both codes be used on the same claim, they should be used, according to this note.

13.31

<u>No, there is an **Excludes1** note</u> indicating that these codes cannot be used together.

Find code M05.611. First, check for any notes under M05.6. There are none. Next, check for notes under M05, because any notes under M05 will apply to all M05 codes. There is an **Excludes1** note under M05 that lists I00. Therefore, I00 cannot be used with any of the M05 codes.

13.32

The code used for this diagnosis is <u>M1A.0221</u>.

Did you find *Chronic gout*, code M1A? Did you read the notes under M1A? There is a **"7ᵗʰ character"** note stating that if the condition is with tophus, there should be a 7ᵗʰ character of 1 added. Keeping that in mind, find the code for *Idiopathic chronic gout, elbow* (M1A.02), and then narrow it down to the left elbow (M1A.022). Next, add the 7ᵗʰ character and you get M1A.0221.

13.33

Marsha suffered a fatigue fracture of a vertebra in the thoracic region. Which of the following is the correct way to code an initial encounter for this injury?

_____ M48.44   _____ M48.44A

_____ M48.44XA   _____ M48.440A

13.34

Jan has primary osteoarthritis of her left hand. What is the code for this condition?

M_____

13.35

Mrs. Brady, age 80, fell and fractured her right forearm (the radius and ulna). She has osteoporosis because of her age. She just went to her doctor for the initial treatment of the fracture. Complete the code.

M_____

There's a code for THAT??

W17.3 is for injuries sustained by falling into a swimming pool. However, there is an **Excludes1** note with this code. W17.3 is only for empty swimming pools. If the swimming pool has water in it you need to use W16.0-. But coders, beware – you're not finished yet! There are separate indented codes for striking the water surface, striking the bottom and striking the wall. Seriously, you can look it up.

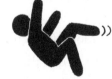

13.33

The correct way to code it is <u>M48.44XA</u>.

Did you read the **"7th character"** note after M48.4? Since this is the initial encounter for the fracture, there should be a 7th character of A added to the code. The code for *Fatigue fracture of vertebra, thoracic region* is M48.44. But this code only has 5 characters, so, we need to add a 6th character. When this situation occurs, a 6th character of X should be added. This gives us the code M48.44XA.

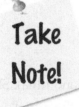

Take Note! Pay attention when using 7th characters with codes. Often times you will need to use one or more X's to make the code seven characters.

13.34

The code for *Primary osteoarthritis of the left hand* is <u>M19.042</u>.

Look for osteoarthritis in the alphabetical index. It is organized by body part. Look for hand. The code is M19.04-. The hyphen indicates that this code needs another character. Look up M19.04 in the tabular list and you'll see that you have three choices: right hand, left hand and unspecified hand. You know that this case involves the left hand, so the correct code is M19.042.

13.35

The correct answer is <u>M80.031A</u>.

If you look up fracture in the alphabetical index, and then forearm, you will be taken to a code that begins with S. This patient has osteoporosis, so look up osteoporosis in the index. You will see "age related" indented under osteoporosis. Under that you see "current pathological fracture" indented. Following the indented codes, find radius or ulna. They both take you to code M80.03. Now find M80.03 in the tabular list and look at the indented codes under it for right forearm: M80.031. This code requires a 7th character (look under M80), which is A, initial encounter for fracture.

Chapter Quiz (Answers in Appendix A)

Let's review some Greek and Latin terms and definitions that we covered in this chapter. Match the definition to the word part.

_____ 13.1 To close	A. dorso
_____ 13.2 Joint fluid	B. phyte
_____ 13.3 Cartilage	C. arthro
_____ 13.4 Back	D. bursa
_____ 13.5 Crookedness	E. spondyl
_____ 13.6 Tendon	F. osteo
_____ 13.7 Bone marrow	G. ankyl
_____ 13.8 Vertebra	H. synov
_____ 13.9 Dissolution; breaking down	I. mal
_____ 13.10 Pore	J. pyro
_____ 13.11 Joint	K. occlusion
_____ 13.12 Dying tissue	L. scoli(o)
_____ 13.13 Arising from; producing	M. teno
_____ 13.14 Bone	N. -lysis
_____ 13.15 Cellular death	O. chondr
_____ 13.16 Sacs in connecting tissue	P. infarct
_____ 13.17 Fire	Q. mye
_____ 13.18 Crooked; stiff	R. necr(o)
_____ 13.19 Bad	S. -genic
_____ 13.20 That which grows	T. por(o)

Match the code to the block title the code is in.

_____ 13.21 M32.0	A.	Infectious arthropathies
_____ 13.22 M94.359	B.	Autoinflammatory syndromes
_____ 13.23 M54.31	C.	Inflammatory polyarthropathies
_____ 13.24 M27.2	D.	Osteoarthritis
_____ 13.25 M99.73	E.	Other joint disorders
_____ 13.26 M47.814	F.	Dentofacial anomalies [including malocclusion] and other disorders of jaw
_____ 13.27 M80.862	G.	Systemic connective tissue disorders
_____ 13.28 M22.01	H.	Deforming dorsopathies
_____ 13.29 M70.42	I.	Spondylopathies
_____ 13.30 M62.221	J.	Other dorsopathies
_____ 13.31 M05.432	K.	Disorders of muscles
_____ 13.32 M41.114	L.	Disorders of synovium and tendon
_____ 13.33 M95.5	M.	Other soft tissue disorders
_____ 13.34 M16.31	N.	Disorders of bone density and structure
_____ 13.35 M86.331	O.	Other osteopathies
_____ 13.36 M65.812	P.	Chondropathies
_____ 13.37 M00.812	Q.	Other disorders of the musculoskeletal system and connective tissue
_____ 13.38 M96.820	R.	Intraoperative and postprocedural complications and disorders of musculoskeletal system, not elsewhere classified
_____ 13.39 M04.1	S.	Periprosthetic fracture around internal prosthetic joint
_____ 13.40 M97.11XA	T.	Biomechanical lesions, not elsewhere classified

14

Diseases of the Genitourinary System

Before we explore the blocks in Chapter 14, please read the **Excludes2** note at the very beginning of the chapter. It lists several conditions in other chapters that should be coded separately but can be used with codes in this chapter.

Let's start with glomerular diseases. The term *glomerular* comes from a Latin word that means "little ball." Medically, it refers to a group of twisted capillaries in the kidney. Look at the first block, **N00-N08** (Glomerular diseases). The

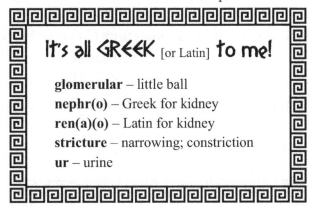

It's all GREEK [or Latin] to me!

glomerular – little ball
nephr(o) – Greek for kidney
ren(a)(o) – Latin for kidney
stricture – narrowing; constriction
ur – urine

first code in this block is N00 *Acute nephritic syndrome*. The term nephritic comes from two word parts: *nephr-* from the Greek meaning kidney and *-ic* means "relating to." So, nephritic means relating to the kidney. As you know, medicine uses both Greek and Latin root words. *Renal* is the Latin root word for kidney.

Read the **Excludes2** note at the beginning of **Block N17-N19** (Acute kidney failure and chronic kidney disease). It specifies some conditions that should be coded separately but can be used with codes in this block. For example, P96.0 *Congenital renal failure* can be coded with N17 *Acute kidney failure*.

Let's look at the word urolithiasis (**Block N20-N23**). You already know two of the parts that make up this word. *Lith-* means stone and *-iasis* means a condition. The new word part is *Ur-*, Greek for urine. So, urolithiasis is the condition of having stones in the urinary tract.

The urolithiasis block is followed by **Block N25-N29**, which covers disorders of the kidney and ureter that are not classified elsewhere.

In medicine, *stricture* is the narrowing of a tube such as the urethra. Find N35 *Urethral stricture* in **Block N30-N39** (Other diseases of the urinary system). This block includes other conditions such as N30 *Cystitis* and N32 *Other disorders of bladder*.

Diseases of male genital organs are found in **Block N40-N53**. It includes diagnoses involving the prostate, testes and penis, and it includes conditions such as male infertility and some male sexual dysfunction.

The terms *mamm(a)(o)* and *mast(o)* both refer to the breast. *Mamm(a)(o)* comes from Latin and *mast(o)* comes from Greek. In **Block N60-N65** (Disorders of breast), find these two codes: N60 *Benign mammary dysplasia* and N60.1 *Diffuse cystic mastopathy*. Did you notice that mammary is based on the Latin root word for breast and mastopathy is based on the Greek word for breast?

Conditions such as N70 *Salpingitis and oophoritis* are included in **Block N70-N77**.

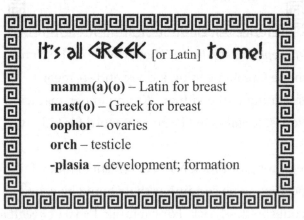

It's all GREEK [or Latin] to me!

mamm(a)(o) – Latin for breast
mast(o) – Greek for breast
oophor – ovaries
orch – testicle
-plasia – development; formation

Let's break it down. Salpingitis, as you learned in Chapter 8, comes from the Greek word *salping-*, for tube, and in this instance is referring to the fallopian tube. So, salpingitis is inflammation of the fallopian tube. *Oophor-* is Greek for ovary. So, oophoritis is inflammation of the ovaries.

Block N80-N98 covers noninflammatory disorders of female genital tract. As you learned in Chapter 9, the prefix *endo-* means within; *metri-* is the lining of the uterus, and *-osis*, of course, means condition. N80 *Endometriosis* is a condition in which uterine cells are growing outside the uterus. Code N81 is *Female genital prolapse*. Prolapse comes from the Latin term and means to fall out of place.

Dysplasia is also found in this block. Dysplasia is made of two terms: *dys-* comes from Greek and means abnormal, while *-plasia*, also from Greek, means development. Therefore, dysplasia is abnormal development.

It's all GREEK [or Latin] **to me!**

cele – tumor; swelling
metra – uterus
oligo – too small; too few
sperm(a) – seed; sperm
vesic(o) – bladder

Remember in Chapter 11 you learned that *cyst-* comes from Greek and means bladder or sac? Well, *vesic(o)-* comes from Latin and also refers to a bladder!

Use these exercises to practice coding in Chapter 14. Hint: for the first three questions, check the Greek/Latin charts at the beginning of this chapter.

14.1

Look at the first block of codes in this chapter, **N00-N08** (Glomerular diseases). What kind of disease is a glomerular disease?

_____ Kidney disease   _____ Bladder disease
_____ Male genital disease   _____ Female genital disease

14.2

The second block of codes in this chapter covers renal tubule-interstitial diseases. What kind of disease is a renal disease?

_____ Kidney disease   _____ Bladder disease
_____ Male genital disease   _____ Female genital disease

14.3

What kind of disease is a nephropathy?

_____ Kidney disease   _____ Bladder disease
_____ Male genital disease   _____ Female genital disease

14.1

A glomerular disease is a <u>kidney disease</u>.

A glomerulus is a group of twisted capillaries or nerve fibers. In this case, it refers to a group of twisted capillaries in the kidney. The word *glomerulus* comes from the Latin for little ball.

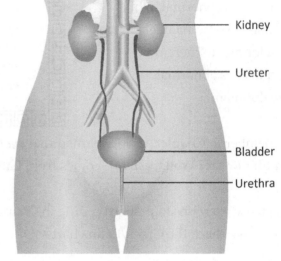

- Kidney
- Ureter
- Bladder
- Urethra

14.2

A renal disease is a <u>kidney disease</u>.

Renal comes from the Latin word for kidney. Renal tubule-interstitial diseases are codes N10-N16.

14.3

Nephropathy means <u>kidney disease</u>.

Did you get stumped on this one? *Nephr-* comes from the Greek word for kidney. So, we have *renal* from Latin and *nephr-* from Greek. It's helpful to remember both of these. And of course *-pathy* means disease.

QUICK QUIZ Answers in Appendix A

_____ 14.1 No or not   *A.* A(n)

_____ 14.2 Slow   *B.* Brady

_____ 14.3 Fast   *C.* Cycl

_____ 14.4 Circle   *D.* Tachy

14.4

Dr. Grey's first patient of the day has a condition called hydronephrosis. The notes say "with renal and ureteral calculous obstruction." Which of these codes will you use?

_____ N13.0   _____ N13.2

_____ N13.1   _____ N13.30

14.5

Dr. Grey's second patient has proteinuria with focal and segmental glomerular lesions. What is the code?

_____ N06.0   _____ N06.2

_____ N06.1   _____ N06.3

14.6

Dr. Grey's next patient has hematuria, blood in his urine. The category for hematuria is:

_____ N01   _____ N03

_____ N02   _____ N04

14.7

Dr. Grey's patient has acute nephritic syndrome with minor glomerular abnormality. Which of these codes will you use?

_____ N00.0   _____ N00.2

_____ N00.1   _____ N00.3

14.8

Dr. Grey's last patient of the morning has acute cystitis with blood in the urine (hematuria). Which code will you use?

_____ N30   _____ N30.01

_____ N30.00   _____ N30.21

14.4

N13.2 *Other hydronephrosis* is the best choice.

Hydronephrosis is the diagnosis for too much water (urine) in the kidney. *Hydro-* means water (in this case it is referring to urine). *Nephro-* means the kidney. *-osis* means condition.

14.5

N06.1 is the correct answer.

Break the word into its parts: *protein-* + *-uria*. *-ur* signifies urine.

14.6

N02 is the correct category. Remember, ICD-10 requires more detail so you must use a subcategory based on the doctor's notes.

If we break the word into its parts, we get *hemat-* = blood, *ur-* = urine, and *-ia* = disease or condition.

14.7

N00.0 is the correct code.

Nephritic pertains to the kidney, and sometimes it is used to mean pertaining to inflammation of the kidney. Break the word into its parts: *nephr-* means kidney; *-ic* means "pertaining to."

14.8

N30.01 is the code for acute cystitis with blood in the urine.

Cystitis is inflammation of the bladder. *Cyst-* is a sac or bladder; in this case it refers to the urinary bladder. You can find cystitis codes in **Block N30-N39** (Other diseases of the urinary system). They are indented under N30 *Cystitis*.

14.9

One of Dr. Grey's patients has vesicoureteral-reflux, code N13.7. Which two body parts are involved? (Hint: break *vesico-*, *ureter-* and *-al* into its terms)

_____ Bladder and kidney   _____ Kidney and ureter

_____ Bladder and ureter   _____ Kidney and urethra

14.10

Look at **Block N20-N23** (Urolithiasis). With your Greek and Latin savvy, what do you think urolithiasis (*ur-*, *lith*, *-iasis*) means?

_____ Pertaining to the ureter and   _____ Any disease in the urinary
      kidney   system

_____ Blockage in the urinary system   _____ Stones in the urinary system

14.11

After an accident Mr. Brown was diagnosed with post-traumatic anterior urethral stricture. Which code will you use? Note: this code requires gender.

_____ N35   _____ N35.010

_____ N35.0   _____ N35.013

14.12

The. Smiths are trying to have a baby, but Mr. Smith has been diagnosed with oligospermia due to infection. Which code will you choose?

_____ N46.121   _____ N46.124

_____ N46.122   _____ N46.125

14.13

Mr. Jones has a condition noted as infected hydrocele. Which code applies to this condition?

_____ N43.0   _____ N43.1

_____ N43.2   _____ N43.3

14.9

Vesicoureteral-reflux is a condition involving the <u>bladder and ureter</u>.

Breaking the word into its parts gives us *vesico-* meaning bladder and *-al* meaning "pertaining to." The ureters are the two tubes that carry urine from the kidneys to the bladder.

14.10

Urolithiasis means <u>stones in the urinary system</u>.

Let's break the word urolithiasis into its parts. *Uro-* refers to the urinary system, *lith-* means stones and *-iasis* means condition.

14.11

<u>N35.013</u> is the correct code.

A urethral stricture is narrowing of the urethra. The urethra is the tube through which urine is released from the body. A *stricture* is a narrowing or constriction.

14.12

<u>N46.122</u> is the code for oligospermia due to infection.

Oligo-, we learned, is the Greek word for small or too few. *Sperma* means seed, and in this case refers to the sperm. Look at code N46 *Male infertility*. There are two major indented codes N46.0 *Azoospermia* (no sperm) and N46.1 *Oligospermia* (too few sperm). An alert coder will see that these two codes are further divided by cause: in this case, it is infection.

14.13

<u>N43.1</u> is the correct code.

Hydro- means water; *-cele* means tumor or swelling. Hydrocele is an accumulation of fluid and occurs in other parts of the body, but in code N43 it refers to the testes, spermatic cord or tunica vaginalis (see the **Includes** note after N43).

14.14

Which code is for a benign cyst of the prepuce?

_____ N47   _____ N47.5
_____ N47.4   _____ N47.8

14.15

Mr. Wrangleman has inflammation of his testicle, which has been diagnosed as orchitis. What is the code for this condition?

_____ N45   _____ N45.2
_____ N45.1   _____ N45.3

14.16

Mammary is a term that refers to the breast. Which of these codes is for mammary duct ectasia of the right breast?

_____ N60.41   _____ N60.81
_____ N60.11   _____ N60.21

14.17

Mastopathy means disease of the breast. Which code is for diffuse cystic mastopathy of the left breast?

_____ N60.82   _____ N60.92
_____ N60.12   _____ N60.22

14.18

Sue has underdevelopment (hypoplasia) of the breast. Which of these codes is best for this condition?

_____ N64.8   _____ N64.82
_____ N64.81   _____ N64.89

14.14

<u>N47.4</u> is for benign cyst of prepuce. The prepuce is the foreskin over the penis.

14.15

<u>N45.2</u> is the code for orchitis.

Orch- is the Greek word for testicles. Remember: N45 is a category which covers both orchitis and epididymitis and therefore is not sufficient as a code. Scroll down to the best detail.

14.16

<u>N60.41</u> is for mammary duct ectasia of right breast.

Mamma- is Latin for breast. Disorders of the breast are found in **Block N60-N65**.

14.17

<u>N60.12</u> is the code for diffuse cystic mastopathy of the left breast.

As is often the case, medical terminology uses both Latin and Greek words to identify the breast. In this case, the Greek word *Masto-* is used. *-pathy* means disease.

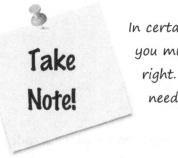

Take Note!

In certain breast disorders you must specify left or right. Sometimes you may need two codes.

14.18

<u>N64.82</u> is for hypoplasia of breast.

Hypoplasia means underdevelopment or incomplete formation of an organ. *Hypo-* comes from the Greek word for under. *-plasia* comes from Greek and means development or formation.

14.19

Paul has a solitary cyst in his left breast. Which code will you choose for this condition?

_____ N60.02   _____ N60.22

_____ N60.12   _____ N60.32

14.20

Maria has been diagnosed with endometriosis of the right ovary, unspecified depth. Which of the following codes will you use for this condition?

_____ N80   _____ N80.101

_____ N80.1   _____ N80.102

14.21

Carolyn's chart indicates complete uterovaginal prolapse. Which one of these codes should you put on the claim?

_____ N81.2   _____ N81.4

_____ N81.3   _____ N81.9

14.22

Martha's fallopian tubes are inflamed. Her doctor says she has acute salpingitis. Which of these codes will you use?

_____ N70.01   _____ N70.11

_____ N70.02   _____ N70.91

14.23

Jane has inflammation of the ovaries. Her doctor has diagnosed chronic oophoritis. Which of these is the correct code?

_____ N70.11   _____ N70.02

_____ N70.12   _____ N70.92

14.19

N60.02 is the best choice.

N60.0 *Solitary cyst of breast* is broken down by right, left and unspecified. N60.02 is for the left breast.

14.20

N80.101 is the code for endometriosis of the right ovary unspecified depth.

Endometriosis is a condition in which uterine cells are growing outside the uterus. *Endo-* means within; *metri-* from the Greek for uterus; *-osis* means condition. Endometriosis is the first code in **Block N80-N98** (Noninflammatory disorders of female genital tract).

14.21

N81.3 *Complete uterovaginal prolapse* is the correct choice.

Prolapse is a condition in which an organ falls out of place. The indented codes under N81 show that there are several codes for female genital prolapse so, as always, choose carefully.

14.22

N70.01 *Acute salpingitis* is the correct choice.

Salpingitis is inflammation of the fallopian tube(s). *Salping-* is the Greek word for tube.

14.23

N70.12 *Chronic oophoritis* (inflammation of the ovaries) is the correct code.

Oophor-, the Greek word meaning "bearing eggs," refers to the ovaries.

Salpingitis and oophoritis sometimes occur together and you can find them listed in the ICD-10 together. For example: code N70.13. Be careful: both oophoritis and salpingitis can be acute (single episode) or chronic (recurring).

14.24

Roger has *Chronic nephritic syndrome with minor glomerular abnormality*. His claim is coded as N03.0. Also on the claim is code N11.0 *Nonobstructive reflux-associated chronic pyelonephritis*. Is it ok to use these two codes together?

_____ Yes, the **Includes** note says to include both
_____ No, the **Excludes1** note says not to code these together

14.25

Maurice has *Chronic obstructive pyelonephritis*. His claim is coded as N11.1. Also on the claim is code N28.85 *Pyeloureteritis cystica*. Is it ok to use these two codes together?

_____ Yes, nothing in the ICD-10 prevents it
_____ No, there is an **Excludes1** note that says not to code these together

14.26

Abe has Stage 1 chronic kidney disease. He also has diabetes mellitus. You decide to code his claim E08.22 *Diabetes mellitus due to underlying condition with diabetic chronic kidney disease* listed first, and N18.1 *Chronic kidney disease, stage 1* listed second. Are you correct?

_____ Yes   _____ No

14.27

You see a claim coded as follows:
        N30.00 *Acute cystitis without hematuria*
        N30.30 *Trigonitis without hematuria*

Is this claim coded correctly?

_____ Yes, there is no problem here
_____ No, N30.30 should be listed first
_____ No, these codes should not be used together

14.24

The correct answer is <u>no, the **Excludes1** note says not to code these together</u>.

Look up N03 *Chronic nephritic syndrome*. Read the **Excludes1** note after this code. It tells you not to use codes that begin with N11 at the same time as codes that begin with N03.

14.25

The correct answer is <u>no, there is an **Excludes1** note that says not to code these together</u>.

To find the answer, look up code N11.1. Now, back up and read the notes under **Block N10-N16** (Renal tubulo-interstitial diseases). There is an **Excludes1** note that says you cannot code N28.85 *Pyeloureteritis cystica* with codes from this block.

14.26

<u>Yes</u>, you are correct. E08.22 is coded first and then N18.1.

The **"Code first"** notes under N18 list E08.22 as a code to use before codes under N18. Under E08.22 there is a **"Use additional code"** note to also identify the stage of chronic kidney disease. Based on these notes, you knew to code E08.22 first and N18.1 second.

14.27

The correct answer is <u>no, these codes should not be used together</u>.

Why? Look up N30.0 and you'll see an **Excludes1** note under it. It excludes using any of the N30.3 codes with N30.0. Cystitis, as you remember, is inflammation of the bladder. Trigonitis is inflammation of the trigone, which is part of the bladder.

QUICK QUIZ Answers in Appendix A

_____ 14.5 Stricture	**A.** Ovaries	
_____ 14.6 Oophor	**B.** Testicle	
_____ 14.7 Cele	**C.** Narrowing	
_____ 14.8 Orch	**D.** Tumor; swelling	

14.28

Dr. Grey has diagnosed Rogelio with "enlarged prostate with lower urinary tract symptoms including nocturia and hesitancy." You see that the claim is coded as shown below. Is this coded correctly?

> N40.1 *Enlarged prostate with lower urinary tract symptoms*
> R35.1 *Nocturia*
> R39.11 *Urinary hesitancy*

_____ Yes, all three should be coded
_____ No, only N40.1 should be coded

14.29

Betty is diagnosed with infertility of tubal origin and incompetence of cervix uteri. Her claim is coded as shown below. Is this coded correctly?

> N97.1 *Female infertility of tubal origin*
> N88.3 *Incompetence of cervix uteri*

_____ Yes, the **Excludes2** note says these can be coded together
_____ No, the **Excludes2** note says these can NOT be coded together

14.30

Aliana has fibroadenosis of her left breast. Look in the alphabetical index under fibroadenosis and decide which code describes this condition.

N_____

14.31

Henrietta has moderate cervical dysplasia. What code describes this condition?

N_____

14.28

The correct answer is yes, all three should be coded.

Find N40.1. The note under this code reads: "Use additional code for associated symptoms, when specified." The associated symptoms for Rogelio are nocturia (urination during the night) and urinary hesitancy. Look up codes R35.1 and R39.11. Each one has a note that says to code first any causal condition such as enlarged prostate.

14.29

The correct answer is yes. The **Excludes2** note says these can be coded together.

Look at code N97.1 and read the **Excludes2** note below N97. As you know, **Excludes2** notes indicate that the two codes are not part of the same condition and both conditions can be listed.

14.30

The complete code is N60.22.

The index directed you to N60.2. From there, it's easy to follow the indented codes to find left breast, which is N60.22. You could also use the blocks at the beginning of this chapter. Find the block for disorder of breast, **Block N60-N65,** and then scan through the block to find the code for fibroadenosis of left breast.

14.31

The complete code is N87.1.

Look up the condition dysplasia in the alphabetical index and find dysplasia of the cervix. The code given is N87.9. But if you look at the indented listings under cervix you will see "moderate" listed as code N87.1. Always look for the most specific code. This is an excellent example of why it's important to check for notes in the chapter that might affect the coding. Did you find the **Excludes1** note after N87?

14.32

Lucy has been having an absence of menstruation. Her doctor notes this as amenorrhea, without giving any further detail. What is the code for this condition?

N_____

14.33

Bob has a kidney stone. His doctor's chart indicates calculus of the kidney. What is the best code for this condition?

N_____

14.34

Mary Lou has a bladder infection. If you break down the conditions below into their roots, which is the term for inflammation of a bladder? Hint: see code N30.

_____ Prostatitis   _____ Nephritis
_____ Cystitis   _____ Orchitis

14.35

What is the complete code for interstitial cystitis (chronic) without hematuria?

N_____

 HOT TIP

It is well worth learning the most common Greek and Latin root words. It's pretty easy and you'll be glad you did when you run across two words that mean the same thing. For example, did you notice that kidney can be referred to as *Renal-* or *Nephro-*? And bladder can be either *Cyst-* or *Vesico-*? And breast can be referred to as *Mammo-* or *Masto-*? Don't you wish they would just pick one and stick with it? Don't worry. With a little practice you'll recognize your Latin and Greek root words and coding will be <u>so</u> much easier.

14.32

The complete code is <u>N91.2</u>.

Look up amenorrhea in the alphabetical index. If the doctor had specified primary amenorrhea, the code would have been N91.0. If secondary, code N91.1.

14.33

The complete code is <u>N20.0</u>.

No math needed here! (Get it? Calculus.) Look up the condition in the alphabetical index. Look through the indented listing until you find kidney. And then look up the code in the tabular list and see if any notes impact the coding.

14.34

<u>Cystitis</u> is the correct term. *Cyst-* is Greek for bladder and *–itis* is inflammation.

14.35

The complete code is <u>N30.10</u>.

Look up cystitis in the index. If you follow the indented list to interstitial (a logical approach), you'll see a note instructing you to look instead for chronic and then interstitial. So, look at the indented listing for chronic, and then interstitial. Once you have the code (N30.10) go to the chapter and check for notes. There are several notes, but none affect this case.

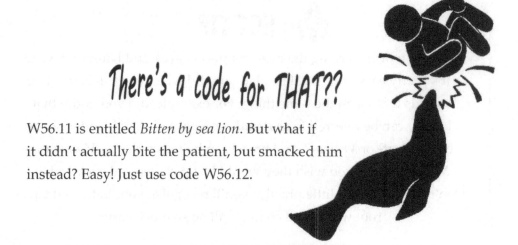

There's a code for THAT??

W56.11 is entitled *Bitten by sea lion*. But what if it didn't actually bite the patient, but smacked him instead? Easy! Just use code W56.12.

Chapter Quiz (Answers in Appendix A)

Referring to the Greek and Latin boxes at the beginning of the chapter match the definition to the word. Some of the Greek and Latin terms from this chapter are bold.

_____ 14.1	Under development	A. **Nephr**itic
_____ 14.2	Uterine cells growing outside uterus	B. Oligo**sperm**ia
_____ 14.3	Abnormal development	C. Hypo**plasia**
_____ 14.4	Low sperm count	D. **Orch**itis
_____ 14.5	Comes from Latin word for kidney	E. **Masto**pathy
_____ 14.6	Term for kidney disease	F. **Uro**lithiasis
_____ 14.7	Pertaining to the kidney	G. **Mamma**ry
_____ 14.8	Inflammation of the ovaries	H. Dys**plasia**
_____ 14.9	Involving the bladder and ureter	I. **Ren**al
_____ 14.10	Inflammation of a testicle	J. **Nephro**pathy
_____ 14.11	Blood in the urine	K. Endo**metri**osis
_____ 14.12	Pertains to the breast	L. **Vesico**ureteral
_____ 14.13	Disease of the breast	M. **Oophor**itis
_____ 14.14	Stones in the urinary system	N. Hema**turia**

Place an A in the blank for each category or subcategory. Place a B in the blank for each code.

_____ 14.15	N13	A. Category or subcategory
_____ 14.16	N48.8	B. Code
_____ 14.17	N25.8	
_____ 14.18	N14.2	
_____ 14.19	N30.2	
_____ 14.20	N18.5	

Match the code to the block title the code is in.

_____ 14.21 N21.1   A. Glomerular diseases

_____ 14.22 N62   B. Renal tubule-interstitial diseases

_____ 14.23 N45.2   C. Acute kidney failure and chronic kidney disease

_____ 14.24 N13.721   D. Urolithiasis

_____ 14.25 N87.1   E. Other disorders of kidney and ureter

_____ 14.26 N28.81   F. Other diseases of the urinary system

_____ 14.27 N70.13   G. Diseases of male genital organs

_____ 14.28 N35.010   H. Disorders of breast

_____ 14.29 N04.2   I. Inflammatory diseases of female pelvic organs

_____ 14.30 N18.3   J. Noninflammatory disorders of female genital
                                tract

_____ 14.31 N99.510   K. Intraoperative and postprocedural complications
                                and disorders of genitourinary system, not
                                elsewhere classified

Indicate all appropriate notes for each code.

14.32 N17.0 ____ ____ ____   A. **Includes**

14.33 N41.3 ____ ____   B. **Excludes1**

14.34 N64.1 ____ ____ ____   C. **Excludes2**

14.35 N28.0 ____ ____   D. **"Use additional code"**

14.36 N04.0 ____ ____ ____ ____   E. **"Code first"**

14.37 N30.11 ____ ____ ____   F. **"Code also"**

14.38 N11.1 ____ ____ ____ ____

14.39 N91.0 ____ ____

15

Pregnancy, Childbirth and the Puerperium

There are four types of notes at the beginning of Chapter 15 in your ICD-10. There's a generic note, a **"Use additional code,"** an **Excludes1** and an **Excludes2**.

The generic note instructs coders to use these codes only on maternal records and never on newborn records. It goes on to specify that codes from this chapter should be used with conditions related to or aggravated by the pregnancy, childbirth, or by the puerperium (period following childbirth) due to either maternal causes or obstetric causes.

The generic note also defines the gestational trimesters, which are counted from the first day of the last menstrual period. The trimesters are defined as:
1st trimester – less than 14 weeks 0 days
2nd trimester – 14 weeks 0 days to less than 28 weeks 0 days
3rd trimester – 28 weeks 0 days until delivery

The **"Use additional code"** note at the beginning of the chapter says to also use a code from category Z3A, *Weeks of gestation*, to identify the specific week of the pregnancy. You will find category Z3A in the last chapter of the ICD-10, between Z36 and Z37.

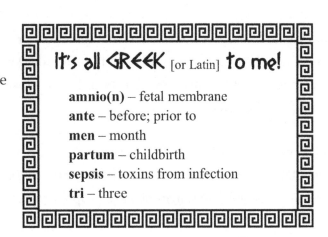

It's all GR€€K [or Latin] to me!

amnio(n) – fetal membrane
ante – before; prior to
men – month
partum – childbirth
sepsis – toxins from infection
tri – three

The **Excludes1** note says you may not use a code from Z34 *Encounter for supervision of normal pregnancy* with any of the codes in this chapter.

Excludes2 says you may use codes for mental and behavioral disorders associated with the puerperium (F53), obstetrical tetanus (A34), postpartum necrosis of pituitary gland (E23.0) and puerperal osteomalacia (M83.0) with codes from this chapter.

Take Note!

Excludes1 means NOT!
In other words the two conditions indicated cannot be coded at the same time.
Excludes2 means TOGETHER!
The condition excluded should be given a different code and you may use the two codes at the same time.

The first block in this chapter covers pregnancies with abortive outcomes. They include O00 *Ectopic pregnancy* and O03 *Spontaneous abortion*, among others.

When there is a high risk pregnancy and supervision is provided you will need a code from **Block O09** (Supervision of high risk pregnancy). The block has only one category, but note that it has many indented codes, which indicate first the reason for the supervision and then the current trimester.

Block O20-O29 covers other maternal disorders predominantly related to pregnancy. Find this block and read the **Excludes2** note. It tells you that codes in the ranges O30-O48 and O98-O99 should be listed separately and can be used with codes from this block.

When there are complications of labor or delivery, you will use codes from **Block O60-O77**. Some of the complications are O60 *Preterm labor*, O63 *Long labor* and O64 *Obstructed labor due to malposition and malpresentation of fetus*.

Block O80-O82 (Encounter for delivery) is one of the simplest blocks in the entire ICD-10. It consists of only two categories: O80 *Encounter for full-term uncomplicated* *delivery* and O82 *Encounter for cesarean delivery without indication*. There are no indented codes, so the three-character code is sufficient. **Block O85-O92 is** dedicated to conditions occurring after delivery.

Now let's work some exercises involving codes from this chapter.

15.1

Mrs. Jones had her first baby and had a full-term uncomplicated delivery. The new coder used both O80 and Z34.00. Is this correct?

_____ Yes, Z34.00 indicates the outcome of the delivery
_____ No, Z34.00 cannot be used with O80

15.2

Read the notes at the beginning of Chapter 15 in the ICD-10. Can the codes in this chapter be used for newborns?

_____ Yes   _____ No

15.3

You are reviewing a claim completed by the new coder. She has used both codes O20.0 and O30.011. Can these two codes be used together?

_____ Yes, because there is an **Excludes2** note which allows this
_____ No, because there is an **Excludes1** note which prohibits this

15.4

Which code is for an incomplete spontaneous abortion without complications?

_____ O03.1   _____ O03.3   _____ O03.4

15.5

Which of these codes is for a classical hydatidiform mole?

_____ O01.1   _____ O01.0   _____ O01.9

15.1

The correct answer is <u>no, Z34.00 cannot be used with O80</u>.

Look at the beginning of Chapter 15. There is an **Excludes1** note covering the Z34 codes. This tells you that you cannot code O80 and Z34.00 together. Now, look under O80 and find the **"Use additional code"** note. It informs you to use Z37.0 to indicate the outcome of the delivery.

15.2

<u>No</u>, the codes in this chapter cannot be used for newborns.

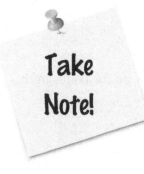

Take Note!

The first note at the beginning of this chapter instructs you to use these codes only for maternal records and never for newborn records.

15.3

The correct answer is <u>yes, there is an **Excludes2** note.</u>

Just beneath code O20 is an **Excludes2** note mentioning codes O30-O48.

15.4

<u>O03.4</u> is the correct code.

The codes for spontaneous abortions begin with O03. Turn to this code and notice that the indented codes are organized by other conditions related to the spontaneous abortion.

15.5

<u>O01.0</u> is the correct choice.

15.6

Which of these codes is for a right tubal pregnancy without intrauterine pregnancy?

_____ O00.1 _____ O00.101 _____ O00.11

15.7

Which of the following is not a type of ectopic pregnancy indented in the ICD-10 under code O00?

_____ Ovarian _____ Abdominal
_____ Vaginal _____ Tubal

15.8

Which code is for hemorrhage specified as due to threatened abortion?

_____ O20 _____ O20.8
_____ O20.0 _____ O20.9

15.9

Dr. Grey's patient has been diagnosed with puerperal sepsis. Which code should you use?

_____ O85 _____ O86.1
_____ O86 _____ O86.8

15.10

Sue Ellen's chart indicates polyhydramnios during her first trimester with a single fetus. Which code will you use?

_____ O40.1 _____ O40.1XX1
_____ O40.1XX0 _____ O40.1XX9

15.6

<u>O00.101</u> is the correct answer. Tubal pregnancy is a type of ectopic pregnancy.

Note that O00.1 is never a complete code because there are indented codes below it.

15.7

<u>Vaginal</u> is not a type of ectopic pregnancy indented under O00.

The types of ectopic pregnancies indented under code O00 are:
O00.0 *Abdominal pregnancy*; O00.1 *Tubal pregnancy*; O00.2 *Ovarian pregnancy*; O00.8 *Other ectopic pregnancy*; O00.9 *Ectopic pregnancy, unspecified*

15.8

The answer is <u>O20.0</u>.

The other choices are incorrect because O20 is the category and can't be used as a code, O20.8 is for "other" and O20.9 is for "unspecified."

15.9

<u>O85</u> *Puerperal sepsis* is the correct answer.

Puerperal sepsis is an infection contracted during or following childbirth. *Sepsis* is based on the Greek word for infection.

15.10

The answer is <u>O40.1XX0</u>.

Polyhydramnios is an excess of amniotic fluid in the amniotic sac. *Poly-* means much or many; *hydr-* means water or fluid; *-amnios* refers to the amniotic fluid. Codes indented beneath O40 are organized by trimester. There is a note beneath O40 stating that these codes require the use of a 7th character. It states that for single gestations the 7th character should be 0. Because the original code (O40.1) has four characters you must add two Xs to be able to put the 7th character in the correct place.

15.11

What code will you choose for eclampsia complicating the pregnancy during the third trimester?

_____ O15.0   _____ O15.02
_____ O15.00   _____ O15.03

Ante- and *post-* are common prefixes in the English language today. Let's look at the medical application of these prefixes.

15.12

Which word means before childbirth?

_____ Antepartum   _____ Postpartum

15.13

Which word means after childbirth?

_____ Antepartum   _____ Postpartum

15.14

Turn to the O99 codes near the end of this chapter in the ICD-10. You might expect O99 to be the last codes, but notice there are O9A codes. Which of the following are the indented codes for O9A?

_____ Malignant neoplasms   _____ Physical abuse
_____ Sexual abuse   _____ Psychological abuse
_____ Injury, poisoning and certain other   _____ All of these
         consequences of external causes

15.15

Look at code O9A.112. If the patient has a malignant neoplasm complicating her pregnancy during the second trimester, should you use code O9A.112 only, or should you also use a code for the neoplasm?

_____ Use only code O9A.112   _____ Also use a code for the neoplasm

15.11

The correct choice is <u>O15.03</u>.

Eclampsia is in category O15 with several indented codes. Now, look at code O14 covering pre-eclampsia. As the Latin prefix *pre-* suggests, it can lead to eclampsia.

15.12

<u>Antepartum</u> means before childbirth.

Ante- = prior to; *-partum* = childbirth.

15.13

<u>Postpartum</u> means after childbirth.

Post- = after; *-partum* = childbirth.

15.14

The correct answer is <u>all of these</u>.

The long ICD-10 description for code O9A is *"Maternal malignant neoplasms, traumatic injuries and abuse classifiable elsewhere but complicating pregnancy, childbirth and the puerperium."* This code includes many things that can complicate a pregnancy. Look at your ICD-10 and you'll see malignant neoplasms, injury, poisoning and certain other consequences of external causes, physical abuse, sexual abuse and psychological abuse.

15.15

When using O9A.112, <u>also use a code for the neoplasm</u>.

The **"Use additional code"** note after O9A.1 instructs you to use an additional code to identify the specific neoplasm.

15.16

Notice that O99 also includes complications of pregnancy. If alcohol use is complicating a pregnancy, should a code from O99 be added to the claim?

_____ Yes, there is a code for alcohol use complicating pregnancy

_____ No, there is not a code for alcohol use complicating pregnancy

15.17

Now, let's look at O98. If the patient has viral hepatitis complicating her pregnancy during the first trimester, which of these codes should be used?

_____ O98   _____ O98.4

_____ O98.41   _____ O98.411

15.18

Sally has an amniotic fluid embolism following a left tubal pregnancy. Which of the following is the correct way to code this?

_____ O00.102, O08.2

_____ O00.102, O08.2 followed by O88.11

_____ O00.102, O88.11 followed by O08.2

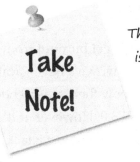

The most descriptive, detailed code is always the one that should be used.

15.16

<u>Yes, there is a code for alcohol use complicating pregnancy</u>.

Code O99.31 covers *Alcohol use complicating pregnancy, childbirth, and the puerperium*. Find this code and notice that it is further indented to specify the time period: trimester, childbirth or puerperium.

15.17

Code <u>O98.411</u> describes the condition in the most detail, therefore it is the one that should be used.

15.18

<u>O00.102, O08.2</u> is the correct way to code amniotic fluid embolism following a left tubal pregnancy.

Start with the ectopic pregnancy code, O00.102. There is a **"Use additional code"** note pointing to the O08 codes. O08.2 is for embolism following ectopic pregnancy, and amniotic fluid embolism is listed as included in this code. O88.11 has an **Excludes1** note saying do NOT use this code with O08.2 (it is just below code O88). Therefore, only O00.102 and O08.2 should be used.

There's a code for THAT??

Most people get burnout from time to time (that's why we have vacations) but who knew there was a code for that? It's Z73.0. However, if it's not actual burnout, but just a lack of relaxation and leisure, use code Z73.2.

15.19

Tonya has pre-existing hypertensive heart disease (without heart failure) complicating her pregnancy. She is in her third trimester. Which is true?

_____ The hypertensive heart disease should be coded first (I11.9) followed by the pregnancy (O10.113)

_____ The pregnancy should be coded first (O10.113) followed by the hypertensive heart disease (I11.9)

15.20

Sonya has a high risk pregnancy because of her history of infertility and the doctor is supervising her progress carefully. She is in her second trimester. Complete the code.

O_____

15.21

Herlinda has developed salpingo-oophoritis during her pregnancy. Complete the code for salpingo-oophoritis that occurs during the third trimester of pregnancy.

O_____

15.22

Maria is having a baby and developed an infection called placentitis in her third trimester. Complete the code for Maria's condition.

O_____

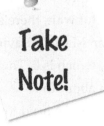

Take Note!

With **"Use additional code"** notes, the code with the note is the primary code and the **"Use additional code"** is the secondary code.

15.19

The pregnancy should be coded first (O10.113), followed by the hypertensive heart disease (I11.9).

If you look up the hypertensive heart disease code (I11.9), you'll see that there are no notes regarding pregnancy. However, if you look up the pregnancy code (O10.113), there is a **"Use additional code"** note regarding the use of I11 codes.

15.20

O09.02 is the code for *Supervision of pregnancy with history of infertility, second trimester*.

O09 (Supervision of high risk pregnancy) is the second block listed. Just look through the **O09** codes until you find the specific code that applies.

15.21

O23.523 is the code for *Salpingo-oophoritis in pregnancy, third trimester*.

Find pregnancy in the alphabetical index. There are many entries under pregnancy, most of which are listed under "complicated by." Look at the indented entries under "complicated by" until you find salpingo-oophoritis, which is O23.52-. The "-" means that at least one more digit is needed. In this case it's the specific trimester. Be sure and look up the code in the tabular list.

15.22

The correct answer is O41.1430.

Look for placentitis in the alphabetical index. The index will direct you to code O41.14. In the tabular list, this code has indented codes that list the trimester. Maria is in her third trimester, so the code to use is O41.143. But wait, there's more! There are instructions after code O41 regarding a 7th character. Maria is having a single baby, so use the 7th character code for single gestation, which is 0. The complete code is now O41.1430. NOTE: read the information about the 7th characters carefully. They state that 0 is for single gestations. 1-9 are used to identify the fetus in cases of multiple gestations.

Chapter Quiz (Answers in Appendix A)

Match the definition to the Greek or Latin word part. Feel free to refer to the Greek and Latin box at the beginning of the chapter.

_____	15.1	Before; prior to	A.	tri
_____	15.2	Fetal membrane	B.	men
_____	15.3	Childbirth	C.	ante
_____	15.4	Three	D.	sepsis
_____	15.5	Month	E.	partum
_____	15.6	Toxins from infection	F.	amnio(n)

Fill in the first letter of codes in each chapter.

_____	15.7	Endocrine system	A or B
_____	15.8	Pregnancy	C or D
_____	15.9	Perinatal period	E
_____	15.10	Nervous system	F
_____	15.11	Digestive system	G
_____	15.12	Eye and adnexa	H
_____	15.13	Neoplasms	I
_____	15.14	Respiratory system	J
_____	15.15	Circulatory system	K
_____	15.16	Mental and behavioral	L
_____	15.17	Skin and subcutaneous tissue	M
_____	15.18	Musculoskeletal system	N
_____	15.19	Genitourinary system	O
_____	15.20	Certain infectious diseases	P

Match the code to the block title the code is in.

_____ 15.21	O23.11	A. Pregnancy with abortive outcome
_____ 15.22	O72.1	B. Supervision of high risk pregnancy
_____ 15.23	O09.71	C. Edema, proteinuria and hypertensive disorders in pregnancy, childbirth and the puerperium
_____ 15.24	O10.313	D. Other maternal disorders predominantly related to pregnancy
_____ 15.25	O9A.219	E. Maternal care related to the fetus and amniotic cavity and possible delivery problems
_____ 15.26	O03.1	F. Complications of labor and delivery
_____ 15.27	O46.013	G. Encounter for delivery
_____ 15.28	O80	H. Complications predominantly related to the puerperium
_____ 15.29	O89.1	I. Other obstetric conditions, not elsewhere classified

Indicate all appropriate notes for each code.

15.30 O29.41 _____ _____ _____ _____	A. **Includes**
15.31 O32.1 _____ _____ _____ _____ _____	B. **Excludes1**
15.32 O12.11 _____ _____ _____	C. **Excludes2**
15.33 O30.012 _____ _____ _____ _____	D. **"Use additional code"**
15.34 O03.2 _____ _____ _____ _____	
15.35 O34.513 _____ _____ _____ _____ _____	E. **"Code first"**
15.36 O36.111 _____ _____ _____ _____ _____	F. **"Code also"**
15.37 O35.4 _____ _____ _____ _____ _____ _____	G. **"7ᵗʰ character"**
15.38 O09.32 _____ _____ _____	
15.39 O43.233 _____ _____ _____ _____	

16

Certain Conditions Originating in the Perinatal Period

This chapter begins with some important notes. Let's take a look.

The first note tells you that codes in this chapter are never to be used on maternal records. These codes are to be used with newborn records only.

The **Includes** note instructs you to use the codes in this chapter for conditions that have their origin in the fetal or perinatal period (before birth through the first 28 days after birth), even if morbidity occurs later. The **Excludes2** note lists several conditions that should be coded separately but can be used with codes in this chapter.

There's another valuable note at the beginning of the first block (**P00-P04**). It instructs you to use these codes when the listed maternal conditions are the cause of illness that originated before birth or during the first 28 days after birth.

It's important to understand that the organization of codes changes not only from chapter to chapter, but also from one block to another. For example, **Block P05-P08** (Disorders of newborn related to length of gestation and fetal growth). Codes P05.00 through P07.18 are organized by weight of the newborn, while codes P07.20 through P07.39, are organized by completed weeks.

The word neonatal, based on a combination of Greek and Latin words (see box), refers to the first few weeks after birth. **Block P09** (Abnormal finding on neonatal screening) is one of the smallest blocks in the ICD-10. It contains only one code. However, notice that there is both a **"Use additional code"** and an **Excludes2** note associated with this code.

If an injury occurs during birth, use a code from **Block P10-P15** (Birth trauma). Browse through these codes and you will see various injuries that can occur during birth. Notice that they are listed by body part.

The root word forming the medical term congenital comes from Latin meaning "born together" or "present at birth." For example, code P23 *Congenital pneumonia* is in **Block P19-P29** (Respiratory and cardiovascular disorders specific to the perinatal period).

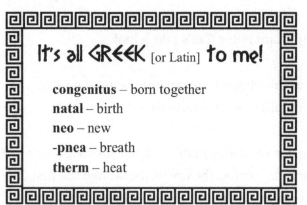

It's all GREEK [or Latin] to me!

congenitus – born together
natal – birth
neo – new
-pnea – breath
therm – heat

Notice the notes at the beginning of the next block, **P35-P39** regarding infections. The first note explains that this block is for infections acquired in the uterus, during birth via the umbilicus, or during the first 28 days after birth. The second note is an **Excludes2** listing some conditions that should be reported separately but that can be billed together with codes in this block.

At the beginning of **Block P50-P61** (Hemorrhagic and hematological disorders of newborn), there's an **Excludes1** note listing codes that cannot be used at the same time as codes in this block.

Hypothermia is a new term from this chapter that is easy to figure out based on two Greek roots. *Hypo-* means under or reduced and *-thermia* means heat. So, hypothermia means below normal body temperature. It is in **Block P80-P83** (Conditions involving the integument and temperature regulation of newborn).

Another block with only one code is **P84** (Other problems with newborn), and it comes with an **Excludes1** note listing codes that cannot be used with it.

This chapter, like many others, has a catch-all block at the end, listing other disorders originating in the perinatal period for conditions not categorized elsewhere.

Let's practice working with the terminology and codes in this chapter.

16.1

The title of this chapter is Certain Conditions Originating in the Perinatal Period. What does perinatal mean?

_____ Prior to birth   _____ Around birth   _____ After birth

16.2

Can codes in Chapter 16 be used with maternal records?

_____ Yes   _____ No

16.3

Based on the Greek and Latin roots (see box), what does neonatal mean?

_____ The last few weeks before birth

_____ During birth

_____ The first few weeks after birth

16.4

Based on the Greek and Latin roots (see box), what does congenital mean?

_____ Present at birth

_____ Occurring prior to birth

_____ Occurring after birth

There's a code for THAT??

If **ze** patient **vas** exposed to **ze** damaging sunlight, use code X32. But **vait**!
Tanning beds and sunburn have their own codes.

16.1

The perinatal period is the period <u>around birth</u>.

Peri- = near. *-natal* = birth. The perinatal period is immediately before or immediately after birth.

16.2

<u>No</u>, the codes in this chapter are not to be used with maternal records.

The note at the beginning of the chapter indicates that the codes in this chapter are for use only with newborns, not with the mothers.

16.3

Neonatal means <u>the first few weeks after birth</u>.

Neo- = new. *-natal* = birth. The neonatal period is the first few weeks after birth.

16.4

Any condition that is congenital was <u>present at birth</u>.

Examples of congenital conditions in this chapter are P23 *Congenital pneumonia*, and P35 *Congenital viral diseases*.

QUICK QUIZ *Answers in Appendix A*

_____ 16.1	Tells you that the codes should never be used at the same time	*A.* Etiology/manifestation
_____ 16.2	Says you must use an additional code, but they can be listed at the same time	*B.* **Excludes1** note
_____ 16.3	Gives examples of content in a category	*C.* **Excludes2** note
_____ 16.4	Tells you that the underlying condition should be coded first	*D.* **Includes** note

---

16.5

You see a claim with a diagnosis of P03.4 *Newborn affected by Cesarean delivery*.
Under which block will this code appear?

_____ **P00-P04** (Newborn affected by maternal factors and by complications of
          pregnancy, labor, and delivery)
_____ **P05-P08** (Disorder of newborn related to length of gestation and fetal
          growth)
_____ **P09** (Abnormal findings on neonatal screening)
_____ **P10-P15** (Birth trauma)

16.6

Look at the codes in the birth trauma block, **P10-P15**. What two words are included
in almost every description in this block?

_____ Birth accident
_____ Birth injury
_____ Near birth
_____ Perinatal damage

16.7

You see a claim with only code listed: P09 *Abnormal findings on neonatal screening*
listed. Can this code be used by itself?

_____ Yes   _____ No

16.8

A newborn has respiratory issues. Under which block of codes will this diagnosis
fall?

_____ **P09** (Abnormal findings on neonatal screening)
_____ **P10-P15** (Birth trauma)
_____ **P19-P29** (Respiratory and cardiovascular disorders specific to the perinatal
          period)
_____ **P35-P39** (Infections specific to the perinatal period)
_____ **P50-P61** (Hemorrhagic and hematological disorders of newborn)

16.5

P03.4 appears in block **P00-P04** (Newborn affected by maternal factors and by complications of pregnancy, labor, and delivery).

16.6

The two words <u>birth injury</u> are included in almost every description of the birth trauma block.

The definition of trauma is "a physical injury or wound caused by an external force." The major categories listed are intracranial laceration and hemorrhage, central nervous system, scalp, skeleton, and peripheral nervous system.

16.7

<u>Yes</u>, P09 can be used by itself.

Why? There is not a **"Use additional code"** note after P09. Remember, the additional codes notes require you to add another code or codes to further identify signs, symptoms and conditions associated with that code. Since there is no **"Use additional code"** note after P09, you can use it by itself.

16.8

Respiratory disorders fall under **Block P19-P29** (Respiratory and cardiovascular disorders specific to the perinatal period).

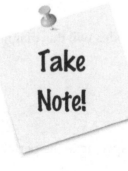

Take Note!

The alphabetical index is a great way to find codes, but the smart coder will also consult the tabular listing (chapters) for notes which will guide you in making the right choice.

16.9

A newborn has been diagnosed with intracranial nontraumatic hemorrhage. Under which block of codes will this diagnosis fall?

_____ P09   _____ P10-P15   _____ P19-P29
_____ P35-P39   _____ P50-P61

16.10

A newborn has stage 1 necrotizing enterocolitis. In which block of codes will you find this diagnosis?

_____ P70-P74   _____ P76-P78   _____ P80-P83
_____ P84   _____ P90-P96

16.11

Dr. Grey's tiny newborn patient has a diagnosis of hypothermia. There are no additional notes on the chart. Which block contains this diagnosis?

_____ P70-P74   _____ P76-P78   _____ P80-P83
_____ P84   _____ P90-P96

16.12

A newborn has noninfective neonatal diarrhea. Complete the code.

P_____

There's a code for THAT??

Remember codes W56.11 and W56.12, involving an unfortunate encounter with a sea lion? Well, there's more! W56.2 is _Contact with orca_ (killer whales); W56.4 is _Contact with shark_; and W56.5 is _Contact with other fish_. And that's just for starters!
Check out all of them at W56.

16.9

Intracranial nontraumatic hemorrhage falls into **Block <u>P50-P61</u>**.

The word hemorrhage is your clue. Look for code P52 *Intracranial nontraumatic hemorrhage of newborn*.

16.10

Stage 1 necrotizing enterocolitis is in **Block <u>P76-P78</u>**.

The correct code is P77.1 *Stage 1 necrotizing enterocolitis in newborn*. Stage 1 necrotizing enterocolitis is a digestive disorder. As you learned in Chapter 11, *entero-* means the intestines; *colo-* refers to the colon and *-itis*, as you know, means inflammation.

16.11

Hypothermia of newborn, unspecified is in **Block <u>P80-P83</u>**.

It is code P80.9 *Hypothermia of newborn, unspecified*. Hypothermia involves temperature regulation. Therefore, you'll find it in this block.

16.12

The complete code is <u>P78.3</u> *Noninfective neonatal diarrhea*.

Start by looking in the alphabetical index for diarrhea. Now, look for neonatal (noninfectious), and you will see it is code P78.3. Now that you know the code you'll want to look in the tabular list and read any notes associated with it.

Another way to find the code is to look under **Block P76-P78** (Digestive system disorders of newborn). Then find P78 *Other perinatal digestive system disorders* and then, indented beneath that, P78.3 *Noninfective neonatal diarrhea*.

16.13

Dr. Grey has determined that the newborn was affected by its mother's condition called oligohydramnios. Complete the code.

P_____

16.14

A newborn was experiencing transient tachypnea. Complete the code for this condition.

P_____

16.15

A newborn has an extremely low birth weight: 605 grams. Complete the code for this condition.

P_____

There's a code for THAT??

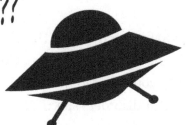

Was your patient injured while making a forced landing with her spacecraft? Code V95.42 has her back!

ICD-10 has our astronauts covered for sure – but please be specific in your coding! For example, if the injury was due to a spacecraft crash, use V95.41; if due to a collision, use V95.43; V95.44 if due to a fire and V95.45 for explosion.

Alert! If the issue was caused by a prolonged stay in a weightless environment such as a spacecraft simulator, that's altogether different! That's code X52.

16.13

The code for newborn affected by maternal oligohydramnios is <u>P01.2</u>.

Oligohydramnios is a maternal condition in which there is not enough amniotic fluid. You will find codes for it in Chapter 15.

Look for this in the alphabetical index under newborn, and then follow this progression: affected by > maternal > oligohydramnios. This will give you code P01.2. And then, of course, look up the code in its own chapter for notes that might affect it.

You could also peruse **Block P00-P04** (Newborn affected by maternal factors and by complications of pregnancy, labor, and delivery).

16.14

The code for *Transient tachypnea of newborn* is <u>P22.1</u>.

According to the root words in Appendix B, *tachy-* means fast and *-pnea* is from the Greek meaning breath or breathing. Tachypnea means rapid breathing. Transient means that the condition is not consistent or that it went away.

How do you find tachypnea? There are two ways: 1) Find it alphabetically in the index, and then look for newborn. Go to the chapter, find the code and check for notes. 2) Or, you can read through the block of codes for respiratory and cardiovascular disorders specific to the perinatal period.

16.15

The complete code for a newborn with a low birth weight of 605 grams is <u>P07.02</u>.

Extremely low birth weight diagnoses are listed in **Block P05-P08** (Disorders of newborn related to length of gestation and fetal growth). Code P07.02 covers birthweights ranging from 500 to 749 grams, so your patient falls within this range. To look this up in the alphabetical index follow this progression: Low > birthweight > extreme > with weight of > 500-749 grams. Then as always, look up the code in the tabular list to check for notes.

Chapter Quiz (Answers in Appendix A)

Fill in the first letter of codes in each chapter.

_____	16.1	Neoplasms	A or B
_____	16.2	Mental, behavioral, and neurodevelopmental disorders	C or D
			D
_____	16.3	Diseases of the circulatory system	E
_____	16.4	Pregnancy, childbirth and the puerperium	F
_____	16.5	Diseases of the digestive system	G
_____	16.6	Congenital malformations, deformations and chromosomal abnormalities	H
			I
_____	16.7	Certain infectious and parasitic diseases	J
_____	16.8	Diseases of the musculoskeletal system and connective tissue	K
			L
_____	16.9	Injury, poisoning and certain other consequences of external causes	M
			N
_____	16.10	Blood and blood forming organs	O
_____	16.11	Diseases of the nervous system	P
_____	16.12	Certain conditions originating in the perinatal period	Q
			R
_____	16.13	Endocrine, nutritional and metabolic diseases	S or T
_____	16.14	Diseases of the respiratory system	
_____	16.15	Diseases of the genitourinary system	
_____	16.16	Diseases of the ear and mastoid process	
_____	16.17	Diseases of the skin and subcutaneous tissue	
_____	16.18	Symptoms, signs and abnormal clinical and laboratory findings	

Indicate all appropriate notes for each code.

16.19 P23.0 ____ ____ ____ ____	A. **Includes**
16.20 P04.11 ____ ____ ____ ____	B. **Excludes1**
16.21 P25.0 ____ ____	C. **Excludes2**
16.22 P58.4 ____ ____ ____ ____ ____	D. **"Use additional code"**
16.23 P00.4 ____ ____ ____	E. **"Code first"**
16.24 P05.2 ____ ____ ____	F. **"Code also"**
16.25 P09 ____ ____	
16.26 P03.2 ____ ____ ____	
16.27 P24.01 ____ ____ ____ ____	
16.28 P91.0 ____ ____ ____	
16.29 P39.1 ____ ____ ____ ____	

Match the code to the block title the code is in.

____ 16.30 P13.2	A.	Newborn affected by maternal factors and by complications of pregnancy, labor, and delivery
____ 16.31 P78.0	B.	Birth trauma
____ 16.32 P04.3	C.	Respiratory and cardiovascular disorders specific to the perinatal period
____ 16.33 P36.4	D.	Infections specific to the perinatal period
____ 16.34 P84	E.	Hemorrhagic and hematological disorders of newborn
____ 16.35 P72.1	F.	Transitory endocrine and metabolic disorders specific to newborn
____ 16.36 P24.11	G.	Digestive system disorders of newborn
____ 16.37 P92.3	H.	Other problems with newborn
____ 16.38 P54.0	I.	Other disorders originating in the perinatal period

17

Congenital Malformations, Deformations and Chromosomal Abnormalities

All of the conditions in this chapter are conditions that exist at birth. It's important to know that codes in Chapter 17 are not to be used on maternal or fetal records. The very first note tells you this. The second note is an **Excludes2**, which lists a block of codes in Chapter 4 that can be used with codes in this chapter, but must be listed separately.

You will notice that the blocks in this chapter are arranged primarily by body part. The last two blocks are entitled "Other congenital malformations" and "Chromosomal abnormalities, not elsewhere classified."

Find code Q02 *Microcephaly*. Looking at the parts of this term, we see *micro-* which means small, and *-cephaly* which refers to the head. The diagnosis for a child born with an abnormally small head is microcephaly. You find this code in **Block Q00-Q07** (Congenital malformations of the nervous system). These codes include conditions for the brain and spinal cord.

Codes Q10 - Q15 are for the eye, Q16 and Q17 are for the ear, and Q18 is for the face and neck. These make up **Block Q10-Q18** (Congenital malformations of eye, ear, face and neck). An **Excludes2** note at the beginning of this block lists several Q codes that can be used with codes in this block, but should be listed separately.

Ophthalmos comes from the ancient Greek word for eye. In code Q11 *Anophthalmos, Microphthalmos and Macrophthalmos* you will see various conditions using this root word. The term **an**ophthalmos means an absence of one or both eyes, **micro**phthalmos means small eye, and **macro**phthalmos means an abnormally large eye.

Find **Block Q30-Q34** (Congenital malformations of the respiratory system). Notice that these codes are organized by body part: nose, larynx, trachea and bronchus, and lung. And, as is usually the case, the last code is a catch all for "other."

Block Q35-Q37 (Cleft lip and cleft palate) also has important notes at the beginning.

The codes in **Block Q38-Q45** (Other congenital malformations of the digestive system) are generally organized by body part beginning with tongue, mouth and pharynx followed by esophagus, upper alimentary tract, small intestine, large intestine, gallbladder, bile ducts and liver, and other.

Congenital malformations of genital organs are found in **Block Q50-Q56**. These

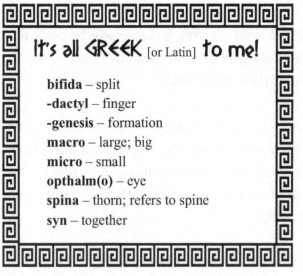

It's all GREEK [or Latin] **to me!**

bifida – split
-dactyl – finger
-genesis – formation
macro – large; big
micro – small
opthalm(o) – eye
spina – thorn; refers to spine
syn – together

codes are organized with the female codes first, followed by the male codes and finally Q56 *Indeterminate sex and pseudohermaphroditism*. Find the **Excludes1** note that lists some diagnoses that cannot be coded with diagnoses in this block.

The codes in the congenital malformations of the urinary system block, **Q60-Q64**, are organized by body parts beginning with kidney, then renal pelvis and ureter followed by codes for "other."

The next block is **Q65-Q79** (Congenital malformations and deformations of the musculoskeletal system). As you look through this block you will notice that it is mostly organized by body part.

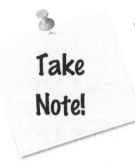

Notice that Q71.0, Q71.1 and many other codes are organized by limb: unspecified, right, left and bilateral. This is a common way for the ICD-10 to list body parts that are on both sides of the body.

These questions will give you some experience in checking notes and understanding how codes are organized.

17.1

In the previous chapter we discussed the term congenital. It means:

_____ Arising from the genital organs
_____ Existing at birth
_____ Having an X and a Y chromosome

17.2

Read the two notes with **Block Q35-Q37** and select the correct statement from the choices below.

_____ Q35.1 and Q87.0 cannot be billed at the same time
_____ Q35.1 and Q30.2 can be billed at the same time
_____ Q35.1 and Q30.2 cannot be billed at the same time

17.3

Can codes in this chapter be used for maternal records?

_____ Yes, some of the codes are designed for maternal records
_____ Yes, but only if used in conjunction with codes from other chapters
_____ No, these codes are not for use with maternal records

17.1

Congenital means <u>existing at birth</u>.

17.2

The correct answer is <u>Q35.1 and Q30.2 can be billed at the same time</u>.

The **Excludes2** note informs you that codes in this **Block Q35-Q37** may be billed with Q87.0, while the "**Use additional code**" note instructs you that it is ok to bill Q30.2 when you bill codes in this block.

17.3

<u>No, these codes are not for use with maternal records</u>.

Why not? A note at the beginning of this chapter informs you that codes in this chapter are not for use with maternal records.

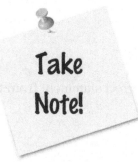

Codes in this chapter are for use <u>only</u>
for conditions existing at birth.

QUICK QUIZ *Answers in Appendix A*		
_____ 17.1 Before or prior to	*A.*	Post
_____ 17.2 After or behind	*B.*	Ante
_____ 17.3 Alongside of	*C.*	Epi
_____ 17.4 Upon or over	*D.*	Para

We already learned the word parts for the next four questions. Open your ICD-10 book to the first four major codes in this chapter: Q00, Q01, Q02 and Q03 and identify these conditions.

17.4

The patient has anencephaly, a condition involving the absence of a major portion of the brain. Which is the correct code?

_____ Q00   _____ Q01.1

_____ Q00.0   _____ Q02

17.5

The patient's diagnosis is occipital encephalocele. Which code is the appropriate choice for this condition?

_____ Q01.0   _____ Q01.1

_____ Q01.2   _____ Q01.8

17.6

The patient has been diagnosed with microcephaly. Which code is the appropriate choice for this condition?

_____ Q01   _____ Q02

_____ Q03   _____ Q04

17.7

Dr. Grey's diagnosis is congenital hydrocephalus but she has not added any specific details. What is the appropriate code to use in this situation?

_____ Q03.0   _____ Q03.1

_____ Q03.8   _____ Q03.9

17.4

Q00.0 *Anencephaly* is the correct choice.

Remember that Q00 is a category and not a complete code because there are indented codes. Let's break down the word into its parts: *An-* means not; *encephal-* relates to the head or brain.

17.5

Q01.2 *Occipital encephalocele* is the correct choice.

Encephalocele is a sac-like protrusion of the brain. Look at the word parts: *encephal-* = brain and *-cele* is a suffix that indicates a tumor or swelling.

17.6

Q02 *Microcephaly* is the correct choice.

This is an appropriate code because it does not have indented codes below it. Microcephaly is an abnormally small head. You know these word parts: *micro-* means small; *cephal-* means head or brain.

17.7

Q03.9 *Congenital hydrocephalus, unspecified* is the correct choice.

Hydrocephalus is an abnormal accumulation of cerebrospinal fluid on the brain. You've learned these word parts! *Hydro-* = water (in this case it refers to cerebrospinal fluid); *cephal-* = head or brain.

QUICK QUIZ Answers in Appendix A		
_____ 17.5 Endo	*A.*	Within or inside
_____ 17.6 Extra	*B.*	Passage or pipe
_____ 17.7 Fistula	*C.*	Outside
_____ 17.8 Fissure	*D.*	Groove or deep furrow

17.8

A baby is born with a congenital defect called lumbar spina bifida. The doctor's notes says there is no hydrocephalus. Which code will you use?

_____ Q05.1   _____ Q05.5

_____ Q05.2   _____ Q05.7

17.9

Which is the correct code for a developmental disorder called microphthalmos?

_____ Q11.0   _____ Q11.1

_____ Q11.2   _____ Q11.3

17.10

Which of these codes is for macrophthalmos?

_____ Q11.0   _____ Q11.1

_____ Q11.2   _____ Q11.3

17.11

Which code is for anophthalmos?

_____ Q11.0   _____ Q11.1

_____ Q11.2   _____ Q11.3

17.12

Look at the block of codes for cleft lip and cleft palate (**Q35-Q37**). Do these codes include an associated malformation of the nose?

_____ Yes, these codes include an associated malformation of the nose

_____ No, an additional code should be used for an associated malformation of the nose

17.8

Q05.7 is the correct code. The diagnosis is lumbar spina bifida without hydrocephalus.

Spina bifida is Latin for split spine.

17.9

Q11.2 *Microphthalmos* is the correct answer.

Microphthalmos means small eye. As is common with medical terms, look for the small words that make up the big word. *Micro-* = small; *-ophthalmos* refers to the eye.

17.10

Macrophthalmos is an abnormally large eyeball. It is listed as code Q11.3.

Look at the word parts: *Macro-* means large or big; *-ophthalmos* refers to the eye.

17.11

Anophthalmos, Q11.1, is the condition of an absence of one or both eyes.

As you know, the prefix *an-* or *a-* means not or no; *-ophthalmos* refers to the eye.

17.12

The correct answer is no, an additional code should be used for an associated malformation of the nose.

Why? You'll find the reason at the notes at the top of the block for cleft lip and cleft palate. There is a "**Use additional code**" note that instructs you to use an additional code for associated malformation of the nose.

17.13

Take a quick look at the code descriptions in the block of codes **Q38-Q45** covering other congenital malformations of the digestive system. How are the codes within this block organized?

_____ Alphabetically by condition

_____ By body part

_____ By seriousness of the condition

17.14

Look at the code descriptions in **Block Q60-Q64** (Congenital malformations of the urinary system). Which organ in the urinary system is listed the most?

_____ Kidney   _____ Bladder

_____ Ureter   _____ Urethra

17.15

Dr. Grey has diagnosed her patient with bilateral renal agenesis. Which of these codes will you select for this condition?

_____ Q60   _____ Q60.0

_____ Q60.1   _____ Q60.2

17.16

You need to look up a code for the doctor's diagnosis of a congenital malformation of the musculoskeletal system. How are the code descriptions arranged in this block of codes (**Q65-Q79**)?

_____ Alphabetically by condition

_____ By body part

_____ By seriousness of the condition

17.13

The codes in the block entitled Other congenital malformations of the digestive system are organized <u>by body part</u>.

The organization is head to toe (well, for the most part): tongue, mouth and pharynx; esophagus; upper alimentary tract; small intestine; large intestine; other intestine; gallbladder, bile ducts and liver; and other digestive system.

17.14

The <u>kidney</u> has the most codes in this block.

17.15

<u>Q60.1</u> *Renal agenesis, bilateral* is the best choice.

Renal agenesis is the failure of one or both kidneys to develop. **Renal** is from the Latin referring to the kidneys. If *a-* means no and *-genesis* means formation, then agenesis means no formation.

17.16

The code descriptions in this block are arranged <u>by body part</u>.

Have you noticed a trend? Although not always the case, many of the codes within a block are organized by body system.

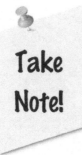

You're ahead of the game knowing that codes are often arranged by body part. Many body parts that are paired, such as eyes, ears, arms and legs, are often arranged by left, right, bilateral and unspecified. In some cases, however, ICD-10 does not have a code for left or right.

Take Note!

17.17

What is the last block of codes in the congenital malformations, deformations and chromosomal abnormalities chapter?

_____ Congenital malformations of the urinary system

_____ Other congenital malformations

_____ Congenital malformations and deformations of the musculoskeletal system

_____ Chromosomal abnormalities, not elsewhere classified

17.18

Dr. Grey records her patient's diagnosis as trisomy 21, translocation. Which code is the best choice?

_____ Q90.0   _____ Q90.1

_____ Q90.2   _____ Q90.9

17.19

A baby is born with a congenital cataract. What is the correct code?

_____ Q12.0   _____ Q12.8

_____ Q12.1   _____ Q12.9

17.20

A baby is born with a congenital pancreatic cyst. Which code describes this condition?

_____ Q45.0   _____ Q45.2

_____ Q45.1   _____ Q45.3

There's a code for THAT??

Are they freckles or are they spots? Be specific, please!
ICD-10 wants you to use L81.2 for _Freckles_ and different codes
for other kinds of spots. For example, see L81.3 for
Café au lait spots (light brown birthmarks).

17.17

The last block of codes in this chapter covers **Q90-Q99** (<u>Chromosomal abnormalities, not elsewhere classified</u>).

17.18

<u>Q90.2</u> is the best choice.

Remember the Greek and Latin roots *tri-* meaning three and *mono-* meaning one? <u>Tri</u>somy is a condition in which there are three instances of a chromosome instead of the normal two. <u>Mono</u>somy, on the other hand, indicates only one instance of a chromosome.

17.19

The block of codes which include congenital cataract is **Q10-Q18** (Congenital malformations of eye, ear, face and neck). The code is <u>Q12.0</u> *Congenital cataract*.

Cataracts affect the lens of the eyes.

17.20

<u>Q45.2</u> *Congenital pancreatic cyst* is listed under **Block Q38-Q45** (Other congenital malformation of digestive system).

If you looked up pancreas in the alphabetical index it would direct you to "see condition," so you would go to cyst, followed by the body part: pancreas, and then the type: congenital.

QUICK QUIZ *Answers in Appendix A*			
_____ 17.9	Micro	*A.*	Split
_____ 17.10	Macro	*B.*	Small
_____ 17.11	Syn	*C.*	Large
_____ 17.12	Bifida	*D.*	Together

17.21

A baby has a congenital ectopic kidney. What code should you use?

_____ Q63.0   _____ Q63.2
_____ Q63.1   _____ Q63.3

17.22

A baby is born with congenital malformation of the great arteries, specifically atresia of the aorta. What code should you use?

_____ Q25.2   _____ Q25.29
_____ Q25.21   _____ Q25.42

17.23

What is the code for congenital laryngocele?

_____ Q31.5   _____ Q31.2
_____ Q31.3   _____ Q31.1

17.24

A baby is born with hypoplasia of the spinal cord. Which of these codes will you select?

_____ Q06.0   _____ Q06.2
_____ Q06.1   _____ Q06.4

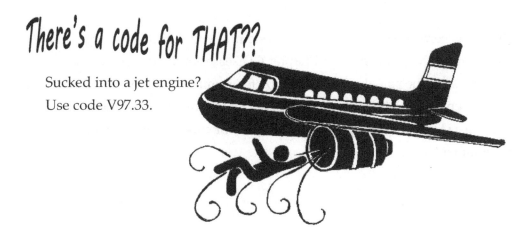

There's a code for THAT??

Sucked into a jet engine?
Use code V97.33.

17.21

Congenital ectopic kidney, code Q63.2 is listed in **Block Q60-Q64** (Congenital malformations of the urinary system).

The kidney is part of the urinary system; however, you will not use one of the codes in Chapter 14 (Diseases of the Genitourinary System) because this condition refers to a newborn and a Q code applies. This rule applies to any diagnosis that is congenital.

17.22

Atresia of the aorta is Q25.29.

Atresia is the condition in which a passage or orifice in the body is abnormally closed or absent. Atresia of aorta is covered in **Block Q20-Q28**.

17.23

Congenital laryngocele is code Q31.3.

A laryngocele is a congenital air sac connected to the larynx. Remember your medical terms: *laryngo-* refers to the larynx and *–cele* means tumor or swelling. The larynx is part of the respiratory system and you'll find any congenital conditions of the larynx in **Block Q30-Q34**.

17.24

Hypoplasia of the spinal cord, Q06.1, is listed in the block for congenital malformations of the nervous system.

The spinal cord is part of the nervous system so you'll find non-congenital conditions of the spinal cord in Chapter 6 Diseases of the Nervous System. Hypoplasia of the spinal cord is incomplete or underdevelopment of the spinal cord. If congenital, it's in **Block Q00-Q07**. Did you break down the word hypoplasia? Recall that *hypo-* means reduced or smaller and *–plasia* means development.

17.25

Dr. Grey's patient was born with an intestinal condition called Hirschsprung's disease. What is the correct code?

_____ Q43.0   _____ Q43.2

_____ Q43.1   _____ Q43.8

17.26

You see a claim with a diagnosis of scrotal transposition. What is the code?

_____ Q55.20   _____ Q55.22

_____ Q55.21   _____ Q55.23

17.27

You coded a claim with a diagnosis of congenital absence of right upper limb. You want to double check that the ICD-10 code is correct. Which of these codes should it be?

_____ Q71.01   _____ Q72.01

_____ Q71.02   _____ Q72.02

17.28

You see a claim with a diagnosis of fused fingers on the left hand. What is the code for this?

Q _____

QUICK QUIZ Answers in Appendix A		
_____ 17.13 -dactyl	A.	Movement
_____ 17.14 -pnea	B.	Formation
_____ 17.15 -genesis	C.	Breath
_____ 17.16 -kinesia	D.	Finger

17.25

Q43.1 is the correct code. Hirschsprung's disease is under **Block Q38-Q45**.

The intestines are part of the digestive system.

17.26

Q55.23 is the correct code. Scrotal transposition is found under **Block Q50-Q56**.

Scrotal transposition is a condition of the male genital organs.

17.27

Q71.01 is the correct code. Congenital absence of right upper limb is listed under **Block Q65-Q79**.

The upper arms are part of the musculoskeletal system. Be sure to check the indented codes under Q71. You should always use the most detailed code!

17.28

The code for *Fused fingers on the left hand* is Q70.02.

If you look up the condition (fused), then find fingers indented beneath it, you will see code Q70.0-. Then you go to the tabular list and find the code for left hand. This code is under the heading Syndactyly. *Syn-* comes from the Greek word for together and *-dactyl* means finger. Syndactyly means that fingers or toes are fused together.

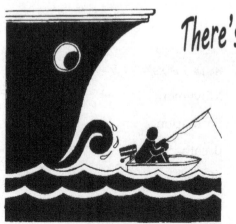

There's a code for THAT??

All smart boaters know to get out of the way of approaching aircraft carriers. But in case the patient didn't move fast enough, use code V94.810 *Civilian watercraft involved in water transport accident with military watercraft.*

17.29

You see a claim with a diagnosis of amyelia – a congenital malformation of the spine. Complete the code.

Q _____

17.30

A baby has a single congenital cyst on her kidney. Complete the code for this condition.

Q6 _____

17.31

You see a claim with a diagnosis of macroglossia. Complete the code for this condition.

Q _____

17.32

Looking at the Chapter-Specific Coding Guidelines for this chapter, which of the following statements is true?

_____ The codes in this chapter should only be used as the primary code
_____ The codes in this chapter should only be used as the secondary code
_____ The codes in this chapter can be used as the primary or the secondary code

17.33

According to the Chapter-Specific Coding Guidelines for this chapter, is this statement True or False?

When there is not a unique code for a malformation, deformation or chromosomal abnormality, additional codes may be used to identify the manifestions that are present.

_____ True   _____ False

17.29

The correct code for *Amyelia* is Q06.0.

If you are unsure of the block, start by looking for amyelia in the alphabetical index. It will direct you to the appropriate code in the tabular list.

17.30

The correct code for a single congenital cyst on the kidney is Q61.01. Notice that ICD-10 does not, in this case, want to know which kidney (right or left).

Since the kidney is part of the urinary system, start by looking in **Block Q60-Q64** (Congenital malformations of the urinary system). You will find Q61.01 *Congenital single renal cyst*. You can also find this in the alphabetical index under cyst > kidney > congenital.

17.31

The correct code for *Macroglossia* is Q38.2.

Find macroglossia in the alphabetical index, and then look for congenital and you can find the code. *Macro-* means large and *-glossia* refers to the tongue.

17.32

The correct answer is the codes in this chapter can be used as the primary or the secondary code.

You'll find this in the first paragraph of the Chapter-Specific Coding Guidelines.

17.33

True. When there is not a unique code for a malformation, deformation or chromosomal abnormality, additional codes may be used to identify the manifestions that are present. You'll find the detailed guidelines in the second paragraph of the Chapter-Specific Coding Guidelines for Chapter 17.

Chapter Quiz (Answers in Appendix A)

Match the definitions to the words. Some of the Greek and Latin terms from this chapter are bold.

_____	17.1	Involves three instances of a chromosome	A. **Micro**cephaly
_____	17.2	Abnormally small head	B. Micr**ophthalmos**
_____	17.3	Absence of one or both eyes	C. Renal **agenesis**
_____	17.4	Existing at birth	D. **Spina** bifida
_____	17.5	Disorder that means small eye	E. Macr**ophthalmos**
_____	17.6	Disorder that means large eye	F. Congenital
_____	17.7	Condition involving the spinal cord	G. An**ophthalmos**
_____	17.8	Kidney(s) fail to develop	H. Monosomy
_____	17.9	Involves only one instance of a chromosome	I. Trisomy

Match the description to the code.

_____	17.10	Occipital encephalocele	A. Q15.0
_____	17.11	Congenital torsion of ovary	B. Q26.0
_____	17.12	Congenital glaucoma	C. Q50.2
_____	17.13	Renal agenesis, unilateral	D. Q24.0
_____	17.14	Congenital subglottic stenosis	E. Q89.01
_____	17.15	Ankyloglossia	F. Q70.32
_____	17.16	Congenital displaced lens	G. Q60.0
_____	17.17	Asplenia (congenital)	H. Q31.1
_____	17.18	Dextrocardia	I. Q12.1
_____	17.19	Webbed toes, left foot	J. Q38.1
_____	17.20	Congenital stenosis of vena cava	K. Q01.2

Use the alphabetical index to find the code for each description.

_____ 17.21   Cleft hard palate with bilateral cleft lip

_____ 17.22   Partial anomalous pulmonary venous connection

_____ 17.23   Longitudinal reduction defect of right femur

_____ 17.24   Hypoplasia of testis and scrotum

_____ 17.25   Agenesis of lung

_____ 17.26   Conjoined twins

_____ 17.27   Displacement of ureter

_____ 17.28   Hypoplasia and dysplasia of spinal cord

_____ 17.29   Atresia of bile ducts

_____ 17.30   Congenital malformation of ear ossicles

_____ 17.31   Whole chromosome trisomy, nonmosaicism (meiotic
                   nondisjunction)

Indicate all appropriate notes for each code.

17.32 Q00.0 _____	A. **Includes**
17.33 Q66.0 _____ _____	B. **Excludes1**
17.34 Q36.0 _____ _____ _____ _____	C. **Excludes2**
17.35 Q92.5 _____ _____ _____ _____	D. **"Use additional code"**
17.36 Q41.1 _____ _____ _____	E. **"Code first"**
17.37 Q05.5 _____ _____ _____ _____	F. **"Code also"**
17.38 Q55.3 _____ _____ _____	
17.39 Q18.2 _____ _____	
17.40 Q95.3 _____ _____	

18

Symptoms, Signs and Abnormal Clinical and Laboratory Findings, Not Elsewhere Classified

Congratulations! You've worked through all the chapters related to specific conditions and body parts. Welcome to Chapter 18 - the R chapter. It is very detailed, with blocks R00 to R94, and is possibly the toughest chapter in the ICD-10! The codes in this chapter are to be used when symptoms are less well defined, or for some other reason a clear diagnosis can't be made.

Coding can be tricky because almost all of the symptoms could be designated "not otherwise specified" (generally codes ending in 8) in the particular chapter covering the affected body part or system. One main reason to use an R code is that the doctor notes that the patient's symptoms could point equally to two or more diseases, or two or more parts of the body.

The detailed note at the beginning of the chapter indicates that the main reasons to use R codes are:

(a) a more detailed diagnosis cannot be made even after all the facts bearing on the case have been investigated;
(b) signs or symptoms that existed at the time of the initial encounter that proved to be transient and whose cause could not be determined;
(c) provisional diagnosis when the patient does not return;
(d) cases referred elsewhere before a diagnosis was made;
(e) a more precise diagnosis was not available for any other reason;
(f) certain symptoms (with supplementary information) that represent important problems in medical care.

The note further instructs you to consult the alphabetical index to determine when to use codes from this chapter and when to use a code from the chapter related to the specific body part or body system.

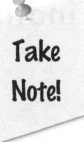

Take Note!

In general, this chapter includes the less well-defined conditions and symptoms that could point equally to two or more diseases or two or more body systems.

The blocks in Chapter 18 are divided this way:

Symptoms and signs
- **R00-R09** Circulatory and respiratory systems
- **R10-R19** Digestive system and abdomen
- **R20-R23** Skin and subcutaneous tissue
- **R25-R29** Nervous and musculoskeletal systems
- **R30-R39** Genitourinary system
- **R40-R46** Cognition, perception, emotional state and behavior
- **R47-R49** Speech and voice
- **R50-R69** General symptoms and signs

Abnormal findings
- **R70-R79** Blood, without diagnosis
- **R80-R82** Urine, without diagnosis
- **R83-R89** Other body fluids, substances & tissues, without diagnosis
- **R90-R94** Diagnostic imaging and in function studies, without diagnosis

Other
- **R97**   Abnormal tumor markers
- **R99**   Ill-defined and unknown cause of mortality

Take a look at **Block R50-R69**. It covers symptoms that could be indicative of any one of many conditions. For example R50 *Fever of other and unknown origin* and R51 *Headache*.

Notice that **Block R70-R79** is for abnormal findings on examination of blood, without diagnosis. Notice they are separated by the type of abnormal findings. It is followed by blocks for examination of urine, examination of other body fluids, substances and tissues, and then diagnostic imaging and in function studies. Following this is **Block R97** for abnormal tumor markers. The codes in these blocks are to be used when abnormal laboratory, imaging, or tumor markers are present but there is no definite diagnosis.

Now, let's practice coding this unusual chapter.

18.1
According to the first paragraph and *Section a* and *Section b* of the Chapter-Specific Coding Guidelines, when do you use the codes in this chapter?

_____ When a definite diagnosis has not been determined
_____ When the sign or symptom is not routinely associated with a diagnosis
_____ In both of these cases

18.2
According to the Chapter-Specific Coding Guidelines, which should be coded first when both the symptom and diagnosis are reported? Example: the patient has tachycardia and the doctor diagnosed it as atrial fibrillation.

_____ The definitive diagnosis
_____ The symptom

18.3
A patient has experienced repeated falls and the doctor has indicated there is risk of future falls. According to the Chapter-Specific Coding Guidelines, is it ok to code R29.6 and Z91.81 together on the same claim?

_____ Yes, these codes can be used together if it is appropriate
_____ No, these codes should never be used together

18.1

The codes in this chapter should be used <u>in both of these cases</u>.

The Chapter-Specific Coding Guidelines tell you to use the codes in this chapter when no diagnosis has been established by the doctor. But it also says that codes in this chapter can be used when there is a definite diagnosis but the signs or symptoms are not routinely associated with the diagnosis.

18.2

The correct answer is <u>the definitive diagnosis code</u> should be sequenced before the symptom code.

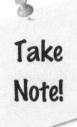

Take Note!

The definite diagnosis should be sequenced before the symptom code.
In addition, signs or symptoms that are routinely associated with a disease process should not be assigned as additional codes, unless otherwise instructed by the ICD-10.

18.3

The codes are R29.6 and Z91.81 and <u>they can be coded together</u>.

R29.6 is for use in this case, in which the patient has experienced repeated falls and a possible medical cause of the fall is being investigated. When there is a history of falling and the patient is at risk for falling in the future, Z91.87 also applies. Both codes can be applicable to one claim.

QUICK QUIZ *Answers in Appendix A*		
_____ 18.1 -algia	*A.*	Disease or condition
_____ 18.2 -rrhea	*B.*	Pertaining to
_____ 18.3 -ary	*C.*	Discharge of pus or fluid
_____ 18.4 -ia	*D.*	Pain

18.4

One of Gabriel's symptoms is dysphasia. How is this coded?

_____ R47.0   _____ R47.02

_____ R47.01   _____ R47.81

18.5

The patient had a urine test and Dr. Watson reports abnormal findings, glycosuria, but she has not made a diagnosis. Which code is for this?

_____ R80   _____ R82

_____ R81   _____ R82.2

18.6

Ms. Fredericksen has a slow heartbeat. Which of these codes will you select?

_____ R00   _____ R00.1

_____ R00.0   _____ R00.2

18.7

Dr. Watson has recorded that the patient has pharyngeal phase dysphagia. Which of these codes applies?

_____ R13.11   _____ R13.14

_____ R13.13   _____ R13.15

18.8

The patient presents with a pallor (paleness) to his skin. What is the symptom code?

_____ R23.0   _____ R23.2

_____ R23.1   _____ R23.3

18.4

<u>R47.02</u> is the correct answer.

Dysphasia is a speech disorder. **Dys-** means bad or difficult and *–phasia* refers to speech.

18.5

<u>R81</u> is the code for glycosuria.

Since there are no codes indented beneath R81 it is an appropriate code to use.

18.6

<u>R00.1</u> is the code for unspecified bradycardia.

Brady-, in Greek, means slow. So, bradycardia means slow heartbeat. You can find slow heartbeat listed beneath R00.1.

18.7

<u>R13.13</u> is for dysphagia, pharyngeal phase.

Dysphagia is difficulty swallowing. As you have learned, *dys-* = bad or difficult and *-phagia* = swallowing. If *-phagia* is preceded by *a-* which means not, then aphagia means not swallowing or unable to swallow.

18.8

<u>R23.1</u> is the code for pallor, a pale color of the skin.

Besides illness there are other possible causes, such as emotional stress, anemia or shock.

QUICK QUIZ *Answers in Appendix A*

_____ 18.5 -dactyl	*A.* split
_____ 18.6 -genesis	*B.* together
_____ 18.7 Syn	*C.* formation
_____ 18.8 Bifida	*D.* finger

18.9

Jim has hypoxemia, an abnormally low level of oxygen in his blood. What is the appropriate code for this?

_____ R09.0   _____ R09.02

_____ R09.01   _____ R09.1

18.10

Dr. Watson has noted the patient's abdominal tenderness in the left lower quadrant. What code applies?

_____ R10.32   _____ R10.814

_____ R10.812   _____ R10.824

18.11

While reviewing a claim you notice it has both codes R22.2 and N63.13. Should both codes be on the same claim?

_____ Yes, because the **Excludes2** note means both can be on one claim

_____ No, because the **Excludes1** note says that both codes should not be on one
       claim

18.12

Which code covers dyslexia, the patient's difficulty in learning to read?

_____ R47.02   _____ R47.01   _____ R49.0

_____ R49.1   _____ R48.0   _____ R06.00

18.13

Hector comes to the doctor with a speech disturbance. The chart says he has aphonia. Which code will you use?

_____ R47.02   _____ R47.01   _____ R49.0

_____ R49.1   _____ R48.0   _____ R06.00

18.9

<u>R09.02</u> *Hypoxemia* is the correct answer.

Hypo- means beneath or below; *ox-* = oxygen; *-emia* = blood.

18.10

<u>R10.814</u> is the correct answer.

18.11

The correct answer is <u>Yes, the **Excludes2** note says that both codes can be on one claim</u>.

Remember: **Excludes2** notes indicate that both codes may be on the same claim, but **Excludes1** notes indicate that they can NOT be on the same claim. In this case, the **Excludes2** note tells you that N63.13 can be on the same claim as R22.2.

18.12

<u>R48.0</u> is the best answer.

Remember the word parts? *Dys-* means difficult or bad; *-lexia* refers to reading. Code R48.0 is for both *Dyslexia and alexia*. The prefix *a-* means not, so alexia is the loss of the ability to read.

18.13

The correct code for aphonia is <u>R49.1</u>.

The prefix *a-* means not and *-phonia* is the root word for voice. Always remember to check for notes that might apply to the code. There is an **Excludes1** note with the category R49 which informs you that you cannot code F44.4 with this category.

QUICK QUIZ *Answers in Appendix A*		
_____ 18.9 Macro	*A.*	refers to spine
_____ 18.10 Opthalm(o)	*B.*	small
_____ 18.11 Micro	*C.*	large; big
_____ 18.12 Spina	*D.*	eye

18.14

Mr. McCarthy has a painful "charley horse" (muscle spasm of the calf). Could this be coded R25.2 *Cramp and spasm* and M62.831 *Muscle spasm of calf?*

_____ Yes   _____ No

18.15

Joseph has a concussion and edema of the cervical spinal cord (S14.0) and the symptom is transient paralysis (R29.5). What is the correct way to code this?

_____ S14.0 and then R29.5   _____ R29.5 and then S14.0
_____ S14.0 only   _____ R29.5 only

18.16

You see a claim with both R79.1 (abnormal coagulation profile) and D68.8 (other specified coagulation defects). Can these two codes be used together on the same claim?

_____ Yes   _____ No

18.17

You see a claim with both code N64.51 (induration of breast - a disorder) and R92.1 (mammographic calcification found on diagnostic imaging of breast - a laboratory finding). Can both of these codes be on the same claim?

_____ Yes, because there is an **Excludes2** note with these codes
_____ No, because there is an **Excludes1** note with these codes
_____ No, because there is an **Excludes2** note with these codes

18.18

Caesar has been diagnosed with hypotension. During the exam his blood pressure reading was low. How should this be coded?

_____ I95.0   _____ I95.0 and R03.1   _____ R03.1

18.14

The correct answer is <u>Yes</u>.

Look up code R25.2 and read the **Excludes2** note. **Excludes2** notes mean the two may be coded together.

18.15

In this case it should be <u>S14.0 and then R29.5</u>.

Looking up S14.0 we find a "**Code also**" note under S14 that mentions R29.5. Looking up R29.5 we find a "**Code first**" note that mentions S14.0. This note tells us to code S14.0 first and then use R29.5.

18.16

<u>No</u>, these two codes cannot be used on the same claim.

Why not? There is an **Excludes1** note under R79.1 that mentions D68.-. This tells you that you cannot use R79.1 with any code that begins with D68.

18.17

The correct answer is <u>yes, there is an **Excludes2** note with these codes</u>.

The **Excludes2** note with N64.5 specifically mentions R92.- and there is an **Excludes2** note at the beginning of Chapter 18 that mentions N64.5.

Excludes2 notes mean the two codes may be used on the same claim.

18.18

The patient has hypotension, so the condition should be coded <u>I95.0</u>.

If you check code R03.1 you will see an **Excludes1** note that excludes the I95.- codes. This means that the two may not be used together. This is a case in which a low blood pressure code does exist (R03.1) as a symptom in this chapter, but it is not necessary because hypotension is the definite diagnosis.

18.19

You see a claim with two codes: The patient's symptom was a wheezing issue called stridor (R06.1) and the doctor's diagnosis was J38.5 (laryngeal spasm). Is it ok for these two codes to be submitted on the same claim?

_____ Yes   _____ No

18.20

Ms. Hernandez's claim shows two malignancies. The first one is coded R18.0 *Malignant ascites* and the second one is coded C56.1 *Malignant neoplasm of right ovary*. Is this the correct order to list these codes?

_____ Yes   _____ No

18.21

You see a claim with two codes: R10.11 (a pain code) and M54.14 (a diagnosis code involving the musculoskeletal system). Is it ok for these two codes to be submitted on the same claim?

_____ Yes   _____ No

18.22

Look at the codes for coma: R40.2. The ICD-10 requires very specific descriptions of the patient's current condition and level of responsiveness. How many coma codes should be used to complete the coma scale when coma is indicated on a claim?

_____ 1   _____ 2   _____ 3   _____ 4

Take Note!

The Chapter-Specific Coding Guidelines about the coma scale also tell you that a code under R40.24 can be used when only the total score is documented and the individual scores are not documented.

18.19

No, codes J38.5 and R06.1 should not be used together.

ICD-10 is very clear on this. There is an **Excludes1** note after R06.1 that excludes J38.5. And, if you look up code J38.5, and then back up to the unindented code J38, you will see an **Excludes1** note that excludes R06.1. These two codes should not be used together.

18.20

No, C56.1 *Malignant neoplasm of right ovary* should be listed first.

Why not? There is a **"Code first"** note after R18.0 that instructs you to code C56 and its indented codes first, and then code R18.0.

18.21

Yes, R10.11 and M54.14 can be billed together.

Why? There is an **Excludes2** note with code R10, the category above R10.11 that mentions M54.-. This means you can use the two together.

18.22

3 coma codes should be used to complete the coma scale.

The note after code R40.2 says that one code from each of the three subcategories R40.21 (whether the eyes are open), R40.22 (the patient's level of verbal response), and R40.23 (the patient's level of motor response) is needed to complete the coma scale.

 HOT TIP

To make sure that you have a good understanding of 7th characters, this is an excellent time to review the information you learned in the Basic Concepts chapter!

Look at the following three scenarios in category R40.2 *Coma* and choose the appropriate code for each.

18.23

Scenario: Patient arrives at emergency department, eyes open to sound.

_____ R40.213A   _____ R40.213X

_____ R40.2132   _____ R40.2133

18.24

Scenario: Patient is oriented upon hospital admission.

_____ R40.225   _____ R40.225X

_____ R40.2252   _____ R40.2253

18.25

Scenario: Patient localizes pain 24 hours or more after hospital admission.

_____ R40.235   _____ R40.235X

_____ R40.2353   _____ R40.2354

There's a code for THAT??

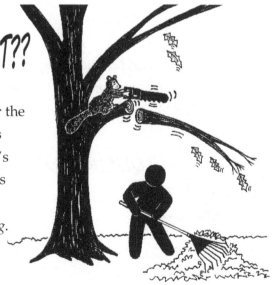

In some cases, ICD-10 has codes for the circumstances under which injuries occur (see Chapter 20). While there's nothing about a crazed squirrel, this incident could be coded Y93.H1 *Activity, digging, shoveling and raking.*

18.23

The correct answer is <u>R40.2132</u>.

How did you decide? The note under R40.21 indicates the need for a 7th character and the appropriate characters available depending on the circumstance. The code for *Coma scale, eyes open, to sound* is R40.213. The 7th character for at arrival to emergency department is 2. This makes the complete code R40.2132.

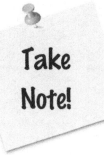

Take Note!

The codes in the coma scale subcategories need 7th characters. Find the note about the 7th character in the ICD-10 in the coma scale codes beneath R40.21, R40.22, R40.23 and R40.24.

18.24

The correct answer is <u>R40.2253</u>.

The code for *Coma scale, best verbal response, oriented* is R40.225. The 7th character for at hospital admission is 3. This makes the complete code R40.2253. Be careful – there is a separate code for hospital admission versus emergency department.

18.25

The correct answer is <u>R40.2354</u>.

The code for *Coma scale, best motor response, localizes pain* is R40.235. The 7th character for 24 hours or more after hospital admission is 4. This makes the complete code R40.2354.

QUICK QUIZ Answers in Appendix A	
_____ 18.13 Congenitus	A. new
_____ 18.14 Neo	B. heat
_____ 18.15 Natal	C. born together
_____ 18.16 Therm	D. birth

18.26

Mrs. Brown presents at the doctor's office with an acute cough. There are no other symptoms. Complete the code.

R_____

18.27

Mrs. Green's symptom is noted as spontaneous ecchymosis on her chart. Complete the code.

R_____

18.28

Mr. Hulk presents with abnormally excessive sweating noted as generalized hyperhidrosis. Complete the code.

R_____

18.29

The laboratory findings indicate glycosuria. Complete the code.

R_____

There's a code for THAT??

In case the patient was injured in the bathroom of their house, it's good to know there's a code for that: Y92.012. But wait! The patient lives in an apartment! Not to worry, there's a code for that: Y92.031. Mobile home? That's Y92.022.

Maybe you think there's not a code if the patient was injured in the bathroom of a reform school. Well, guess again! There's a code for that, too! Y92.152. Just for fun, take a break and check out the place of occurrence codes under Y92.

18.26

The complete code for *Acute Cough* is <u>R05.1</u>.

Look in the alphabetical index for cough. Then find acute, the code is R05.1. As always, look the code up in the tabular list and check for notes. Notice that the **Excludes1** note under R05 says that two types of cough may not be coded here. They are A37.1- (paroxysmal cough due to Bordetella pertussis) and J41.0 (smoker's cough).

18.27

<u>R23.3</u> is the complete code for *Spontaneous ecchymosis*.

Ecchymosis is bleeding beneath the skin resulting in discoloration. Look for ecchymosis in the alphabetical index, and then scan down the indented codes to find spontaneous. The code is R23.3. Find this code in the tabular list and see that **Excludes1** note says not to use this code with a newborn and an **Excludes2** note with the block excludes certain symptoms relating to the breast.

18.28

The complete code for *Generalized hyperhidrosis* is <u>R61</u>.

Hyperhidrosis is abnormally increased sweating. *Hyper-* means increased, *hidros-* refers to sweat and *-osis* means condition. Look up hyperhidrosis in the alphabetical index. Next, scan down and find generalized. The code is R61. In this case, there is a **"Code first"** note but it doesn't apply to this patient. An **Excludes1** note under R61 indicates some L codes that cannot be used with R61.

18.29

The correct answer is <u>R81</u>.

Glycosuria is the condition of having glucose in the urine (*glyco- + -uria*). Look up glycosuria in the alphabetical index. You have a choice between glycosuria and renal glycosuria. In this case, we know we want the one that begins with R as this is for laboratory findings. The code for glycosuria is R81. Now, look up R81 in the tabular listing and notice the **Excludes1** note under code R81 referring to renal glycosuria.

Chapter Quiz (Answers in Appendix A)

Match the definitions to the words. Some of the Greek and Latin terms from this chapter are bold.

_____ 18.1	Loss of the ability to read	A.	Dys**phagia**
_____ 18.2	Abnormally increased sweating	B.	Hypoxemia
_____ 18.3	Difficulty swallowing	C.	**Aphagia**
_____ 18.4	Abnormally low level of oxygen in the blood	D.	**Alexia**
		E.	Hyper**hidros**is
_____ 18.5	Speech disturbance	F.	**Aphonia**
_____ 18.6	Unable to swallow		

Look up each code and fill in the blank with the appropriate 7th character.

_____ 18.7   R40.243 - at hospital admission

_____ 18.8   R40.241 - in the field [EMT or ambulance]

_____ 18.9   R40.233 - 24 hours or more after hospital admission

_____ 18.10   R40.214 – unspecified time

_____ 18.11   R40.222 – at arrival to emergency department

If the code is for a symptom, place an S in the blank. If the code is for a finding, place an F in the blank.

_____ 18.12   R45.83 *Excessive crying of child, adolescent or adult*

_____ 18.13   R88.0 *Cloudy (hemodialysis) (peritoneal) dialysis effluent*

_____ 18.14   R00.2 *Palpitations*

_____ 18.15   R29.810 *Facial weakness*

_____ 18.16   R73.02 *Impaired glucose tolerance (oral)*

Match the code to the description on the right.

_____ 18.17 R19.34	A. Retention of urine that is drug induced
_____ 18.18 R41.2	B. An infant with an idiopathic pulmonary hemorrhage that is acute
_____ 18.19 R94.01	C. Mass and lump with generalized intra-abdominal and pelvic swelling
_____ 18.20 R40.2212	D. Behavior that is compulsive and obsessive
_____ 18.21 R78.71	E. Abdominal rigidity of the left lower quadrant
_____ 18.22 R87.615	F. An erythrocyte sedimentation rate that is elevated
_____ 18.23 R44.1	G. Ecchymoses that is spontaneous
_____ 18.24 R70.0	H. Amnesia that is retrograde
_____ 18.25 R45.850	I. Level of lead in the blood is abnormal
_____ 18.26 R33.0	J. The reason for the visit is obscure due to verbosity and circumstantial detail
_____ 18.27 R46.81	K. Cardiac murmur that is benign and innocent
_____ 18.28 R94.121	L. A fever after a procedure
_____ 18.29 R46.7	M. Cytologic smear of cervix that is unsatisfactory
_____ 18.30 R01.0	N. Mass and lump on the right lower limb with localized swelling
_____ 18.31 R19.07	O. Electroencephalogram [EEG] results are abnormal
_____ 18.32 R22.41	P. Ideations that are homicidal
_____ 18.33 R50.82	Q. Hallucinations of a visual nature
_____ 18.34 R04.81	R. Vestibular function study results are abnormal
_____ 18.35 R23.3	S. No verbal response on the coma scale upon arrival at the emergency department

19

Injury, Poisoning and Certain Other Consequences of External Causes

In this chapter you'll see that some codes begin with S and some begin with T. The S codes are for injuries and are organized by body part, beginning with the head and moving down the body to the foot.

The codes that begin with T encompass a multitude of conditions including burns and corrosions, frostbite, poisoning and complications of surgical and medical care. There are only two injury codes that begin with T: T07 for injuries to multiple body regions and T14 for injury when the body region is not specified. Notice that all the codes in this chapter are for external causes as opposed to illness or conditions covered in the previous chapters.

The ICD-10 instructs you to record not only the nature of the injury, but also the cause of the injury. While the codes in Chapter 19 covers the injury itself, the codes in Chapter 20 will explain the cause of the injury. A note at the beginning of this chapter tells you to use codes from Chapter 20 as secondary to the codes in Chapter 19. This means that you should use the code from Chapter 19 first, followed by the applicable code from Chapter 20.

The note also tells you that some T codes include the cause, so you don't need to use an additional code from Chapter 20 for these. For example, T36 includes the cause (adverse effect of and underdosing of systemic antibiotics) so there is no need to add a code from Chapter 20.

To recap: in most cases, if the diagnosis requires a code from Chapter 19, you will also need a second code from Chapter 20 explaining the cause.

An unusual feature of this chapter is that the burns and corrosions blocks are grouped into a "super-block," **T20-T32** (Burns and corrosions). It is divided this way:

T20-T25 (Burns and corrosions of external body surface, specified by site),
T26-T28 (Burns and corrosions confined to eye and internal organs), and
T30-T32 (Burns and corrosions of multiple and unspecified body regions).
This "super-block" lists some **Includes** notes and an **Excludes2** note that apply to all the burns and corrosions blocks.

Placeholders and 7ᵗʰ characters
Most codes in Chapter 19 require a 7ᵗʰ character, so this is a good time to review this ICD-10 rule. Most often your choices will be A, D or S. However, fractures have additional 7ᵗʰ character choices available.

> **A = initial encounter** – patient is receiving active treatment
> **D = subsequent encounter** – routine care during healing phase
> **S = sequela** – complications of the condition

In the Basic Concepts chapter we discussed placeholders. A placeholder is an X. When a 7ᵗʰ character is needed and the code has fewer than six digits, you will need to add one or more Xs so the 7ᵗʰ character will be in the correct place.

Let's look at some scenarios using 7ᵗʰ characters.
Scenario 1: The patient is diagnosed with a contusion of the scalp and this visit is for active treatment of the contusion. The code is S00.03. That gives you five characters. Now what? Take it step by step. The 7ᵗʰ characters that apply to this code are listed just below S00. You need to choose between A, D and S. The 7ᵗʰ character A is for use when the patient is receiving active treatment for the condition, so A is the correct choice. In order to make the code have seven characters, you must add an X after the 3, so the complete code becomes S00.03XA.

Scenario 2: the patient returns to the doctor for routine follow-up care for an injury of the optic nerve of the left side. The code for this condition is S04.012. The applicable 7ᵗʰ character codes are listed under S04 and consist of A, D, and S. In this case you will choose D, the 7ᵗʰ character for routine follow-up care.

So the complete code is S04.012D. Since the condition code already had six characters and D makes seven, you do not need to add an X.

Scenario 3: Our patient has an unspecified fracture of the upper end of the right ulna and is seeing the doctor for a subsequent encounter for a closed fracture with delayed healing. Start by finding S52.0 *Fracture of upper end of ulna*. Looking at the indented codes we find S52.00 *Unspecified fracture of upper end of ulna* and indented below it is further detail specifying the right ulna, or S52.001. Now, take a look at the list of 7th characters applicable to the S52 codes. Remember, fractures will have more than three choices for 7th character codes. The 7th character would be G (subsequent encounter for closed fracture with delayed healing). This gives you the code S52.001G.

Always check the list of 7th characters that apply to the code you are using. For example, look at S72 *Fracture of femur*. There is a list of 16 letters that can be used as 7th characters. But S72.47 *Torus fracture of lower end of femur* has its own set of 7th characters with just 6 listed.

Let's practice coding in this chapter with the exercises below.

19.1

According to the Chapter-Specific Coding Guidelines, do most codes in this chapter require a 7th character?

_____ Yes, most codes in this chapter require a 7th character
_____ No, most codes in this chapter do not require a 7th character

19.2

Dr. Able diagnosed a patient with a fractured alveolus of the mandible. The code is S02.67. Today's visit was a follow-up due to delayed healing. What is the 7th character?

_____ A   _____ G
_____ B   _____ K
_____ D   _____ S

19.1

The correct answer is <u>yes, most codes in this chapter require a 7th character.</u>

Section a of the Chapter-Specific Coding Guidelines for Chapter 19 goes into detail regarding the use of 7th characters. Be sure to study this section.

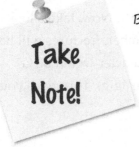

Become a 7th character expert and you're on your way to being best in the field! Incorrect use of 7th characters can get your claim processed incorrectly or possibly denied.

19.2

The correct 7th character for subsequent encounter for fracture with delayed healing is <u>G</u>.

The list of appropriate 7th characters for S02.67 are shown just below S02.

There's a code for THAT??

Falling on ice and snow is common, and the ICD-10 requires you to be very specific. For example, the code for *Fall from stairs and steps due to ice and snow* is W00.1 and the code for *Other fall from one level to another due to ice and snow* is W00.2. If you are not sure, use *Unspecified fall due to ice and snow* (W00.9). Did you notice that these codes require the use of a 7th character?

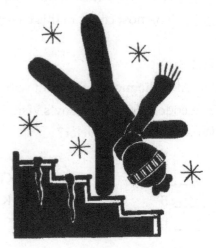

19.3

Juan was in a motorcycle accident. He has some minor contusions and a deep cut
on his left forearm with some nerve damage. Should both the contusions and the
nerve damage be coded? Hint: Read *section b* of the Chapter-Specific Coding
Guidelines, coding of injuries.

_____ Yes, always code all injuries even when they are the same site

_____ No, superficial injuries should not be coded with more severe injuries of the
    same site

19.4

Paola fell out of a tree and has a fracture. The doctor's notes do not indicate
whether the fracture is open or closed. How should this be coded? Hint: read the
notes in *Section c* of the Chapter-Specific Coding Guidelines.

_____ Code as an open fracture   _____ Code as a closed fracture

19.5

This chapter contains codes for burns and corrosions. Are burns and corrosions
considered the same in the ICD-10?

_____ Yes, a burn is a corrosion and a corrosion is a burn

_____ No, burns and corrosions are not the same thing in the ICD-10

19.6

Are burns and corrosions subject to the same guidelines?

_____ Yes, the guidelines are the same for both burns and corrosions

_____ No, the guidelines for burns are different than the guidelines for corrosions

19.7

How should burn codes be sequenced for multiple sites?

_____ Start with the top of the head and move down toward the toes

_____ The code that reflects the highest degree of burn should be listed first

_____ The sites should be coded starting with the least severe to the most severe

19.3

The correct answer is <u>no, superficial injuries should not be coded with more severe injuries of the same site</u>.

The Chapter-Specific Coding Guidelines specify that superficial injuries should not be coded when associated with more severe injuries of the same site.

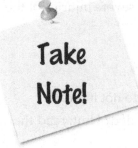

Take Note!

The Chapter-Specific Coding Guidelines also state that when coding multiple injuries, you should list the code for the most serious injury first.

19.4

According to the Chapter-Specific Coding Guidelines, if a fracture is not indicated as open or closed, <u>it should be coded as a closed fracture</u>.

19.5

If you checked the Chapter-Specific Coding Guidelines for coding of burns and corrosions, good for you! You learned that the correct answer is <u>no, burns and corrosions are not the same thing in the ICD-10</u>.

19.6

The correct answer is <u>yes, the guidelines are the same for both burns and corrosions</u>.

19.7

The correct answer is <u>the code that reflects the highest degree of burn should be listed first.</u>

You'll find the instructions in *Section d subsection 1* of the Chapter-Specific Coding Guidelines for sequencing of burn and related condition codes.

> **Take Note!**
> The ICD-10 makes a distinction between burns and corrosions. An injury caused by a heat source such as fire, hot appliance, radiation or electricity is considered a burn. Sunburn is not considered a burn. ICD-10 specifies that chemical burns are considered corrosions.

19.8

Which 7th character should be used for a claim with sequela of burns or corrosions?

_____ A   _____ D

_____ S   _____ A, D or S can be used

19.9

True or False? The Chapter-Specific Coding Guidelines tells you that since there is a Table of Drugs and Chemicals in the ICD-10, you should always code directly from this table. Therefore, you do not need to refer to the tabular list.

_____ True   _____ False

19.10

Which of the following is the guideline to follow when poisoning from multiple drugs is involved?

_____ Code only the major drug ingested

_____ Use as many codes as necessary to describe all drugs ingested

_____ Code the two which were the most consumed

19.11

Which of the following is the proper sequencing of codes when adult or child abuse is involved?

_____ First use the appropriate adult or child abuse code, followed by any mental health or injury codes

_____ First use mental health or injury codes. Use the appropriate adult or child abuse code last

19.8

S is the 7th character used for sequela on burns and corrosions.

Remember that sequela means a follow-up visit. The Chapter-Specific Coding Guidelines *Section d subsection 7* states that S should be used. Also note that *Section d subsection 8* says that A or D should only be used along with S when someone has a current burn and sequela of an old burn at the same time.

19.9

The correct answer is <u>False</u>.

The Chapter-Specific Coding Guidelines instruct you to always refer back to the tabular list and NOT to code directly from the Table of Drugs and Chemicals. Why? Because there are coding notes in the tabular list that need to be considered.

19.10

When multiple drugs are involved, <u>use as many codes as necessary to describe all drugs ingested</u>.

You'll find this instruction in *Section e subsection 2*.

19.11

<u>List first the appropriate adult or child abuse code, followed by any mental health or injury codes</u>.

Section f covers coding for the results of adult and child abuse, neglect and other maltreatment. It states that the appropriate care for adult and child abuse should be listed first, followed by the codes for any mental health or injury.

QUICK QUIZ *Answers in Appendix A*	
_____ 19.1 Sharp or severe	*A.* Chronic
_____ 19.2 Over time	*B.* Acute
_____ 19.3 Bad or difficult	*C.* Polar
_____ 19.4 Opposite in character	*D.* Dys

19.12

According to the notes at the beginning of Chapter 19, should you use an additional code from Chapter 20 with the codes from Chapter 19?

_____ Yes, you should always use a code from Chapter 20 with these codes

_____ Yes, except for the T codes in Chapter 19 that already include the external cause

_____ No, you should never use a code from Chapter 20 with these codes

19.13

Look at blocks **S00-S09** through **S90-S99**. How are they organized?

_____ Alphabetically   _____ By body part

_____ By type of injury   _____ By name of poison

19.14

Notice that all S codes cover injuries. What do T codes cover?

_____ Burns

_____ Burns and poisoning

_____ Certain injuries, burns, poisoning and some other causes

19.15

Melissa sees her doctor for an abrasion of the scalp which was coded as S00.01. There is some infection associated. Which of the following is true?

_____ Only the abrasion code should be used

_____ Only the infection code should be used

_____ Both the abrasion code and the
        infection code should be used

There's a code for THAT??

Paper cuts are annoying, but seriously?
They have their own code? Yes! It's
W26.2 *Contact with edge of stiff paper.*

19.12

The correct answer is <u>yes, except the T codes in Chapter 19 that include the external cause</u>. These do not require an additional external cause code.

The note at the beginning of Chapter 19 says to use secondary codes from Chapter 20 to indicate the cause of the injury. However, some codes in the T section of Chapter 19 already include the external cause; therefore they do NOT require an additional code.

19.13

Blocks **S00-S09** through **S90-S99** are organized <u>by body part</u>.

They start with injuries to the head (**S00-S09**) and continue down the body to injuries to the ankle and foot (**S90-S99**).

19.14

The correct answer is <u>T codes cover certain injuries, burns, poisoning and some other causes</u>.

The S codes are neat and orderly – they are all about injuries to body parts, from the head down. The T codes, well, that's a different story. The T codes have a couple of blocks for injury, one for the effects of a foreign body, several blocks for burns and corrosions, one block for frostbite, one for poisoning, one for toxic effects, two for complications, and a catch-all for "other and unspecified" external causes. To be sure you've coded correctly, it's smart to do a quick scan every time. You will become more familiar with the blocks as you work with them.

19.15

The correct answer is <u>both the abrasion code and the infection code should be used</u>.

The key to this is the **"Code also"** note for **Block S00-S09**. It tells you that you should also code any associated infection for conditions in this block. And don't forget the 7th character! If this is the initial visit, the 7th character A should be used, giving you a final code for the abrasion of S00.01XA.

19.16

Hans saw Dr. Able for superficial frostbite on his nose. What is the correct code for
his second visit to Dr. Able?

_____ T33.02   _____ T33.02D

_____ T33.02A   _____ T33.02XD

19.17

Tommy got a splinter in his left ear. His mom takes him to his doctor. What is the
correct code for Tommy's first visit to the doctor for this condition? Hint: Don't
forget to read the notes.

_____ S00.452   _____ S00.452X

_____ S00.452A   _____ S00.452S

19.18

Mauricio was involved in an accident resulting in a traumatic rupture of his right
eardrum. The emergency room doctor treated him. Which of the following is
correct?

_____ S09.21   _____ S09.21A

_____ S09.21XA   _____ S09.21XS

19.19

Hector fell off his bicycle last month and sustained a puncture wound of his right
breast with no foreign body. He also suffered a fracture of one rib on his right side.
Today he visited his doctor for a follow-up visit. His doctor said he is doing fine.
How will you code this?

_____ S22.31D, S21.031D

_____ S21.031A, S22.31XA

_____ S21.031D, S22.31XD

19.16

The code for a second visit for superficial frostbite of nose is <u>T33.02XD</u>.

The code for superficial frostbite of nose is T33.02. There is a note telling you that a 7th character must be used with this code. Because this is a subsequent encounter you must use a D as the 7th character. That brings it up to only six characters, so you must add an X as a placeholder to bring it up to seven.

19.17

The code for initial visit for superficial foreign body of left ear is <u>S00.452A</u>.

The base code is S00.452, but don't forget about the 7th character. This is an initial visit, so look for the 7th character that indicates initial visit. It's an A. This gives you the complete code: S00.452A.

19.18

The code for emergency room visit for traumatic rupture of right eardrum is <u>S09.21XA</u>.

S09.21 is the code for traumatic rupture of the right ear drum. Notice that this code requires a 7th character. Look at the table for 7th characters. Mauricio was treated in the emergency room and the 7th character for initial encounter is A. But this code still only has six characters, so you must add an X as a placeholder.

19.19

If you got this right, congratulations! It wasn't an easy one. The follow-up visit code is <u>S21.031D, S22.31XD</u>.

Here's the sequence: The code for the puncture wound of the right breast without a foreign body is S21.031. The notes after code S21 say to also indicate the S22.31 code (fracture of a right rib). This means the sequence is S21.031, and then S22.31. A 7th character of D is required for each code because this is a subsequent encounter, this give you S21.031D and S22.31D. The latter code only has six characters, so you must insert an X as a placeholder to get S22.31XD.

19.20

Lee was in a car accident and has a longitudinal fracture of the right patella. What is the code for the initial encounter?

S_____

19.21

Taylor has a nondisplaced fracture of the proximal phalanx of his right thumb. Today's visit is for a subsequent visit involving delayed healing. Complete the code.

S_____

19.22

Henrietta fell while dancing and sustained a strained muscle of her left hip. The doctor is seeing her for late effects from her injury. Complete the code for late effects of the muscle strain.

S_____

19.23

John tripped while jogging and has a displaced fracture of the distal phalanx of his right great toe. Complete the code for a subsequent encounter with nonunion.

S_____

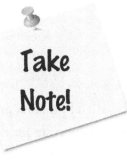

Take Note!

If there is a 7th character available for a code, you must use it.

19.20

The complete code for the initial encounter is <u>S82.021A</u>.

Here's the sequence of steps to the correct code: Look up fracture, traumatic in the alphabetical index and find patella, longitudinal. The code is S82.02-. Find S82.02 in the S chapter of the tabular list. How do you know if this is displaced or nondisplaced? Read the notes under S82. If not indicated on the chart as displaced or nondisplaced, it should be coded as displaced. How do you know if it was open or closed? The notes under S82 say that if not indicated as open or closed it should be coded as closed. This is the initial encounter for closed fracture, so use 7th character A.

19.21

The complete code for subsequent visit with delayed healing is <u>S62.514G</u>.

In the index, find fracture, traumatic, and then thumb, proximal phalange, nondisplaced. The code is S62.51-. Look up the code in the tabular list and find nondisplaced and right thumb on the same code, S62.514. Read the notes under S62. The 7th character you need is G: subsequent encounter for fracture with delayed healing.

19.22

The complete code for late effects of the muscle strain is <u>S76.012S</u>.

In the index, look up injury, muscle, hip, strain. This takes you to code S76.01. Look up this code and then find the left hip, S76.012. Now, read the notes under S76 and find the 7th character for sequela (late effects). The 7th character to use is S.

19.23

The complete code is <u>S92.421K</u>.

In the index find fracture, traumatic, and then find toe, distal phalanx and displaced, S92.42. Look this up in the tabular list and find the code for right great toe, S92.421. Now, check the notes after S92 and find the appropriate 7th character. This is a subsequent visit with nonunion, so the 7th character is K.

19.24

True or False? According to the Chapter-Specific Coding Guidelines, you should never use T07 in an inpatient setting.

_____ True

_____ False

19.25

Most, if not all, of the S codes require a 7th character. Now, flip through the T codes and take a look. Do most of the T codes require a 7th character?

_____ Yes, most of the T codes require a 7th character

_____ No, only a few of the T codes require a 7th character

19.26

Dr. Able removes a foreign body from a child's right ear. It is an initial encounter. Complete the code.

T_____

19.27

Roger has a first degree burn on his left palm. Complete the code for a follow up visit.

T_____

There's a code for THAT??

Yes, there is! W49.01 *Hair causing external constriction*. Wow, talk about a bad hair day.

19.24

The correct answer is <u>False</u>.

Code T07 covers injuries involving multiple body regions. The Chapter-Specific Coding Guidelines say that this code is only to be used in an inpatient setting if information for a more specific code is not available. It probably won't be used often, but it can be used in an inpatient setting.

19.25

The correct answer is <u>yes, most of the T codes require a 7th character</u>.

The vast majority of the T codes require a 7th character using one of these three characters:

A for the initial encounter
D for subsequent encounter
S for sequela

19.26

The initial encounter code is <u>T16.1XXA</u>.

You can find this in the alphabetical index by looking for foreign body, ear. It's best to look up the condition rather than the body part in the alphabetical index. This gives you code T16.-. Now go to the T chapter, which is Chapter 19, and look up T16 in the tabular list and find the code for right ear, T16.1. If you look at the notes under T16, you will see that the 7th character to use for an initial encounter is A. Since the code has only four characters, you must use two placeholder Xs to bring the code up to the required seven characters.

19.27

The follow up visit code is <u>T23.152D</u>.

In the alphabetical index look up burn, palm, left, first degree. This gives you the code T23.152. Now, look up this code in the tabular list, and you can check for notes. Under T23 you will see the note giving you the 7th character. For a subsequent visit, the 7th character is D.

Chapter Quiz (Answers in Appendix A)

Use the alphabetical index to find the code for each description.

_____ 19.1   Abrasion of scalp, sequela

_____ 19.2   Moderate laceration of liver, subsequent encounter

_____ 19.3   Contusion of abdominal wall, initial encounter

_____ 19.4   Open bite of left thumb without damage to nail, subsequent encounter

_____ 19.5   Traumatic rupture of left ear drum, initial encounter

_____ 19.6   Torus fracture of lower end of right femur, subsequent encounter for fracture with delayed healing

_____ 19.7   Nondisplaced fracture of neck of right radius, sequela

_____ 19.8   Puncture wound with foreign body of nose, initial encounter

_____ 19.9   Laceration without foreign body of left shoulder, sequela

_____ 19.10 Fracture of alveolus of right mandible, initial encounter

Indicate all appropriate notes for each code.

19.11 S06.370 ____ ____ ____ ____ ____ ____		A. **Includes**
19.12 S40.812 ____ ____ ____ ____ ____		B. **Excludes1**
19.13 S94.02 ____ ____ ____ ____ ____		C. **Excludes2**
19.14 S33.120 ____ ____ ____ ____ ____ ____		D. **"Use additional code"**
19.15 S63.312 ____ ____ ____ ____ ____ ____		
19.16 S12.040 ____ ____ ____ ____ ____ ____		E. **"Code first"**
19.17 S76.012 ____ ____ ____ ____ ____		F. **"Code also"**
19.18 S21.031 ____ ____ ____ ____ ____ ____		G. **"7ᵗʰ character"**
19.19 S50.852 ____ ____ ____ ____		
19.20 S82.015 ____ ____ ____ ____ ____		

Use the alphabetical index to find the code for each description.

_____ 19.21 Burn of esophagus, initial encounter

_____ 19.22 Anaphylactic reaction to peanuts, subsequent encounter

_____ 19.23 Heat exhaustion due to salt depletion, initial encounter

_____ 19.24 Asphyxiation due to plastic bag, accidental, sequela

_____ 19.25 Burn of second degree of neck, initial encounter

_____ 19.26 Unspecified foreign body in trachea causing
                  asphyxiation, subsequent encounter

_____ 19.27 Leakage of a nephrostomy catheter, initial encounter

_____ 19.28 Foreign body in cornea, right eye, subsequent encounter

_____ 19.29 Burn of first degree of left ear [any part, except ear drum],
                  sequela

_____ 19.30 Superficial frostbite of right ankle, initial encounter

_____ 19.31 Corrosion of second degree of left wrist, sequela

_____ 19.32 Deprivation of water, initial encounter

Indicate all appropriate notes for each code.

19.33 T26.51 ____ ____ ____ ____ ____ ____	A.	**Includes**
19.34 T32.0 ____ ____ ____ ____	B.	**Excludes1**
19.35 T18.110 ____ ____ ____ ____	C.	**Excludes2**
19.36 T36.7X1 ____ ____ ____ ____ ____ ____	D.	**"Use additional code"**
19.37 T20.012 ____ ____ ____ ____ ____	E.	**"Code first"**
	F.	**"7ᵗʰ character"**

If the code includes the cause place a Y in the blank, otherwise place an N.

____ 19.38	T36.0X3		____ 19.40	T20.212
____ 19.39	T33.511		____ 19.41	T37.1X4

20

External Causes of Morbidity

Chapter 20 covers events and circumstances that caused an injury or condition, such as an accident or poisoning. A note at the beginning of the chapter explains that these codes should be used as a second code. The first code will come from the specific chapter that covers the injury itself. Most often that will be Chapter 19: Injury, poisoning and certain other consequences of external causes, codes S00-T88.

For example, a patient was in an automobile accident and broke his shoulder. Intuitively, you might go straight to Chapter 13 which covers the musculoskeletal system of which the shoulder is part. However, that chapter covers *diseases* of the musculoskeletal system and this is an *injury*. So, your first code will come from Chapter 19.

Take Note!

The codes in Chapter 20 should not be used as the primary diagnosis. They are intended to be used as secondary to codes in other chapters.

The Chapter-Specific Coding Guidelines for this chapter say that there is no national requirement to use the codes in Chapter 20. However, there may be state or payer requirements. These codes are most commonly used to provide helpful statistical information.

Codes in this chapter begin with V, W, X and Y. They are grouped into three types: V00-V99 for transport accidents – cars, motorcycles, buses, and other related vehicles; W00-X58 for other external causes of accidental injury such as falling, guns, animals, etc, and X71-Y99 for various other external causes such as war, assault, and medical mistakes. This chapter is very descriptive as to the cause. Remember, ICD-10 instructs you to select the most detailed code possible. Many of these codes require the use of a 7th character.

Block V00-V99 (Transport accidents) is further subdivided into blocks based on the type of transport. These types of transport are pedestrian, pedal cycle rider, motorcycle rider, occupant of three-wheeled motor vehicle, car occupant, occupant of a pick-up truck or van, occupant of heavy transport, bus occupant, other land transport, water transport, air and space transport, and - just in case they missed anything - codes V98-V99 cover "other and unspecified transport."

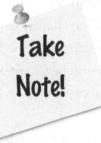

Take Note!

*The transports accident block has many notes. In addition to the standard "**Use additional code**," **Excludes1** and **Excludes2** notes, you'll find additional notes explaining how to use certain specific codes.*

Block W00-X58 covers other external causes of accidental injury due to causes other than transport accidents. Some examples are: **W00-W19** (Slipping, tripping, stumbling and falls), **W20-W49** (Exposure to inanimate mechanical forces), **W50-W64** (Exposure to animate mechanical forces), **X00-X08** (Exposure to smoke, fire and flames), and **X30-X39** (Exposure to forces of nature). You'll see many additional notes to help you narrow down to the most complete code.

The other remaining blocks with X codes are **X71-X83** (Intentional self-harm) and **X92-Y09** (Assault). Notice that both blocks are subdivided by the way the harm was perpetrated, for example, drowning (X71) and handgun discharge (X72).

The first block of exclusively Y codes is **Y21-Y33** (Event of undetermined intent). A note at the beginning of this block instructs you that if there's no documentation that specifies the injury as intentional you should code it as accidental.

The rest of this chapter covers a range of causes, from legal intervention, operations of war, military operations, and terrorism (**Y35-Y38**) to causes as the result of surgical and medical care (**Y62-Y84**) or medical devices (**Y70-Y82**). The last block (**Y90-Y99**) provides supplementary information concerning causes of morbidity. Look through these codes and you will see that many provide for place of occurrence or activity at the time of occurrence, such as Y92.

The ICD-10 provides an index specifically for this chapter. When you need to look up an external cause for an injury, just go to the External Cause of Injuries Index.

This is an unusual chapter. Let's begin to master it with these exercises.

20.1
According to the note in the beginning of the chapter, which two of the following statements are true?

_____ Codes in this chapter should be used as the primary code
_____ Codes in this chapter should be used secondary to another code
_____ Codes in this chapter will most often be used with codes from Chapter 19

20.2
The U codes cover

_____ Injuries due to terrorism
_____ Self-harm injuries
_____ Unspecified causes of injuries
_____ None of the above

20.3
According to the Chapter-Specific Coding Guidelines, what is the national requirement regarding codes in Chapter 20?

_____ These codes are required by the federal government
_____ There is no national requirement to use any of the codes in Chapter 20

20.4
How many external cause codes can you use?

_____ Only one   _____ Two
_____ Three   _____ As many as needed

20.1

The correct answers are:

Codes in this chapter should be used secondary to another code

Codes in this chapter will most often be used with codes from Chapter 19

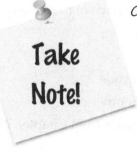

Codes in this chapter are not intended to be used alone. They should be used as secondary codes along with codes from other chapters, primarily (but not always) Chapter 19.

20.2

The answer is None of the above.

There are currently no U codes in the ICD-10. Why? That's a very good question! This letter is being saved for emergency code additions.

20.3

The correct answer is There is no national requirement to use any of the codes in Chapter 20.

While the federal government doesn't require using the External Causes of Morbidity codes, there may be some states or payers that do.

20.4

You should use as many external cause codes as needed.

If more than one external cause code applies to a situation, more than one external cause code should be used. The rule is simple: use as many external cause codes as you need to fully describe the causes.

20.5

Read the note under code Y93 and then answer this question: You see a bill with a Y92 code and a Y93 code listed together. Is this correct?

_____ Yes, both Y92 codes and Y93 codes should be on the same bill

_____ No, Y92 and Y93 codes should never be used together

20.6

Read the section in the Chapter-Specific Coding Guidelines covering multiple external causes. Which of the following statements is true?

_____ External cause codes for terrorism take precedence over all other external cause codes

_____ External cause codes for child and adult abuse take precedence over all other external cause codes

_____ External cause codes for transport accidents take precedence over all other external cause codes

20.7

If a person is injured while changing the tire on an automobile, can a code from **Block V00-V09** be used? Hint: You'll find the answer in the notes below the heading "Pedestrian injured in transport accident".

_____ Yes, the notes say this would be included in **V00-V09**

_____ No, a person changing a tire is not in a transport vehicle

20.8

Read the notes at the beginning of **Block V10-V19** (Pedal cycle rider injured in transport accident). Does this block cover an injury related to the rupture of a bicycle tire?

_____ Yes, the note says pedal cycle tires are included

_____ No, the note says pedal cycle tires are not included

20.5

Yes, both Y92 codes and Y93 codes should be on the same bill.

The note under Y93 tells you to use a place of occurrence code (Y92) with activity codes (Y93).

20.6

The correct answer is external cause codes for child and adult abuse take precedence over all other external cause codes.

The order of precedence for external cause codes is:

Child and adult abuse

Terrorism

Cataclysmic events

Transport accidents

If two or more external causes apply, you should use both but be sure to keep them in this priority order.

20.7

The correct answer is yes, the notes say this would be included in **V00-V09**.

How do you know? An **Includes** note after the heading "Pedestrian injured in transport accident (**V00-V09**)" says to include injury changing a tire on a transport vehicle. It also specifies injury incurred while examining the engine of a vehicle broken down on the side of the road.

20.8

The correct answer is no, the note says it does not include injury due to the rupture of a pedal cycle tire.

Why not? The **Excludes2** note specifies that injury due to rupture of a pedal cycle tire is excluded. It should be coded as W37.0.

20.9

Oscar was the driver of an armored car when it had an accident. Which block of codes should be used?

_____ Occupant of pick-up truck or van injured in transport accident

_____ Occupant of heavy transport vehicle injured in transport accident

_____ Bus occupant injured in transport accident

_____ Other land transport accidents

20.10

Samantha fell from her horse, and the new coder listed her injury under **Block W00-W19** (Slipping, tripping, stumbling and falls). Is this correct?

_____ Yes, this is correct

_____ No, falling from an animal is excluded from this block

20.11

Raj was struck by lightning. Should this be coded in the block covering exposure to electric current, radiation and extreme ambient air temperature and pressure **(W85-W90)**?

_____ Yes

_____ No

20.12

Page through the codes that begin with V. Which of these codes need a 7th character?

_____ V00-V19

_____ V60 only

_____ All V codes

20.9

You should use **Block V60-V69** (<u>Occupant of heavy transport vehicle injured in transport accident</u>) when someone is in an armored car accident.

The **Includes** note at the beginning of this block specifically states that it includes 18 wheelers, armored cars and panel trucks. Did you notice the **Excludes1** note regarding buses and motorcoaches? These are covered in **Block V70-V79**.

20.10

The correct answer is <u>no, falling from an animal is excluded from this block</u>.

The **Excludes1** note at the beginning of this block specifies that V80.- should be used for an injury resulting from falling from an animal.

20.11

The correct answer is <u>no</u>.

Why? There is an **Excludes1** note at the beginning of the block called "Exposure to electric current, radiation and extreme ambient air temperature and pressure." Lightning is listed as excluded. The code for lightning strikes is T75.0-.

20.12

The answer is <u>all V codes should have a 7th character</u>.

The 7th character will come from this list:
A – initial encounter; D – subsequent encounter; S – sequela

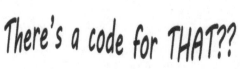

Who knew sewing would warrant
its own code: See Y93.D2.

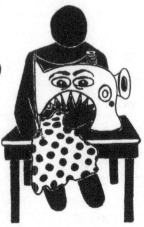

20.13

Page through the codes that begin with W. Which of these codes need a 7th character?

_____ W65-W74

_____ W21 and W 22 only

_____ All W codes

20.14

Page through the codes that begin with X. Which of these codes need a 7th character?

_____ All X codes

_____ X codes X15 and X16 only

_____ None of the X codes should have a 7th character

20.15

Page through the codes that begin with Y. Which of these codes need a 7th character?

_____ Only Y62   _____ None of the Y codes

_____ All of the Y codes   _____ Some, but not all of the Y codes

20.16

William was struck by a baseball. Complete the code for an initial encounter.

W_____

20.17

Hugo was working on his car and accidentally touched the hot engine. What is the code for a subsequent visit for burn by contacting a hot engine? Hint: the word subsequent is your clue.

X_____

20.13

The correct answer is <u>all W codes should have a 7th character</u>.

The 7th character should come from this list:
A – initial encounter; D – subsequent encounter; S – sequela

20.14

The correct answer is <u>all X codes should have a 7th character</u>.

The 7th character should come from this list:
A – initial encounter; D – subsequent encounter; S – sequela

20.15

The correct answer is <u>some Y codes, but not all should have a 7th character</u>.

It is advisable not to guess regarding 7th characters. Take the time to read all the notes and avoid having to re-code a claim.

20.16

The complete code is <u>W21.03XA</u>.

Begin by looking in the External Cause of Injuries Index for Struck by. Look at the indented listing for baseball. This gives code W21.03, so look it up in the tabular list. This category requires use of the 7th character, A, for initial encounter. You will need to add a placeholder X, giving you the complete code W21.03XA.

20.17

The complete code is <u>X17.XXXD</u>.

Look in the External Cause of Injuries Index for burn. Scroll down and find engine (hot). The code is X17. Now, look up X17 in the tabular list and notice that the category does not have any indented codes, so use X17. But, the category requires the use of a 7th character and for subsequent encounter this is D. You need to use three placeholder Xs, giving the complete code X17.XXXD.

20.18

A patient intentionally shot himself with a handgun. The chart indicated attempted suicide. Complete the code for an initial encounter.

X_____

20.19

Maria was injured in a tornado. Complete the code for a subsequent encounter.

X_____

20.20

Jorge was injured while riding his bicycle. He collided with another bicycle in a traffic accident. Complete the code for the initial encounter.

V_____

There's a code for THAT??

If you find yourself being carried by other people and they drop you causing injury, don't worry. You'll be pleased to know that there's a code for that: W04. You'll need to add a 7th character to indicate initial encounter, subsequent encounter or sequela.

20.18

The correct answer is <u>X72.XXXA</u>.

In the External Cause of Injuries Index, find suicide, then firearm, then handgun. This refers you to code X72. Look up this code in the tabular index, look for notes and you will see the 7th characters that are valid for this code. A is for initial encounter. But, that gives you only four characters, so you need three placeholder Xs to make it seven characters long.

20.19

The correct answer is <u>X37.1XXD</u>.

Use the External Cause of Injuries Index and look up tornado (any injury) which is code X37.1. Look this up in the tabular index and notice that the 7th character for subsequent encounter is D. Did you remember to add your placeholders? You need to insert two Xs to get to seven characters.

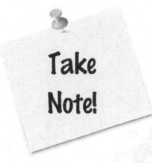

Take Note!

Sometimes you must insert two or more placeholders (X's) to add up to seven characters.

20.20

The correct answer is <u>V11.4XXA</u>.

If you search for bicycle in the External Cause of Injuries Index you find, "see Accident, transport, pedal cyclist." Following this, look down the list for "pedal cycle (traffic)." This gives you V11.4. Or, you could look in the "Pedal cycle rider injured in transport accident" block of Chapter 20 for collision with other pedal cycle in a traffic accident and get to V11.4. Check for notes and remember to add the 7th character A for initial encounter. That brings you to only five characters, so you'll need to insert two X's to make A the 7th character.

Chapter Quiz (Answers in Appendix A)

Match the code to the block title the code is in.

_____ 20.1	V86.12XA	A.	Pedestrian injured in transport accident
_____ 20.2	V47.11XS	B.	Pedal cycle rider injured in transport accident
_____ 20.3	V24.2XXS	C.	Motorcycle rider injured in transport accident
_____ 20.4	V95.25XD	D.	Occupant of three-wheeled motor vehicle injured in transport accident
_____ 20.5	V78.5XXA		
_____ 20.6	V92.01XD	E.	Car occupant injured in transport accident
_____ 20.7	V18.0XXS	F.	Occupant of pick-up truck or van injured in transport accident
_____ 20.8	V98.3XXA		
_____ 20.9	V38.5XXD	G.	Occupant of heavy transport vehicle injured in transport accident
_____ 20.10	V58.0XXA		
_____ 20.11	V64.7XXS	H.	Bus occupant injured in transport accident
_____ 20.12	V05.02XA	I.	Other land transport accidents
		J.	Water transport accidents
		K.	Air and space transport accidents
		L.	Other and unspecified transport accidents

Indicate all appropriate notes for each code.

20.13	W20.1 _____ _____ _____	A.	**Includes**
20.14	V80.42 _____ _____ _____ _____	B.	**Excludes1**
20.15	V28.4 _____ _____ _____ _____ _____	C.	**Excludes2**
20.16	W16.521 _____ _____ _____	D.	**"Use additional code"**
20.17	V57.1 _____ _____ _____ _____ _____	E.	**"Code first"**
20.18	V03.91 _____ _____ _____ _____ _____	F.	**"Code also"**
20.19	X93 _____ _____ _____	G.	**"7th character"**

Use the External Cause of Injuries Index to find the code for each description.

_____ 20.20 Bitten by dog, subsequent encounter

_____ 20.21 Fall from chair, initial encounter

_____ 20.22 Struck by basketball, initial encounter

_____ 20.23 Motorcycle passenger injured in collision with car in traffic accident, initial encounter

_____ 20.24 Exposure to tanning bed, subsequent encounter

_____ 20.25 Assault by airgun discharge, sequela

_____ 20.26 Contact with hot toaster, initial encounter

_____ 20.27 In-line roller-skater colliding with a stationary object, subsequent encounter

_____ 20.28 Overdose of radiation given during therapy

_____ 20.29 Overexertion from prolonged static or awkward postures, subsequent encounter

_____ 20.30 Exposure to ignition of highly flammable material, initial encounter

_____ 20.31 Contact with knife, undetermined intent, sequela

_____ 20.32 Legal intervention involving injury by tear gas, bystander injured, subsequent encounter

_____ 20.33 Car passenger injured in collision with pick-up truck in traffic accident, initial encounter

_____ 20.34 Exposure to excessive natural heat, sequela

_____ 20.35 Private garage of single-family (private) house as the place of occurrence of the external cause

_____ 20.36 Passenger on bus injured in collision with railway train or railway vehicle in traffic accident, sequela

21

Factors Influencing Health Status and Contact with Health Services

Here we are at the Z codes. Did you think you'd ever get here?

The Z codes represent reasons for encounters. They are provided for occasions when circumstances other than a disease, injury or external cause in all the previous chapters are recorded as "diagnoses" or "problems." In other words, these are not codes for diagnoses of specific problems. There are two main ways this applies:

     1) When a person receives health services such as a wellness exam, home health care, to donate an organ, receive a vaccination or discuss a problem which is not a disease or injury, and

     2) When a circumstance or problem is influencing the person's health but is not a current illness or injury. For example, a person in an abusive situation in which no injuries have occurred, or exposure to a suspected contagious disease.

You will find some new terms in this chapter. A status code indicates that a patient is either a carrier of a disease or has the residual of a past disease or condition. A history code indicates a past medical condition that no longer exists. You will find a list of codes for both in the Chapter-Specific Coding Guidelines. Screenings make up a large segment of Z codes. It is an early detection test for disease in a patient who shows no signs of an illness or condition.

The first block, **Z00-Z13,** covers examinations. These are codes for general exams, newborn and infant exams, routine child exams, examination of potential organ donor, eye and hearing exams, dental exams and cleaning, medical observation for suspected diseases and conditions ruled out, and other types of encounters for exams and screenings. When you need a code for a routine exam regardless of the body system involved, this is the place to look!

Your first thought might be to go to Chapter 14 (N codes) for a routine breast exam, or Chapter 16 (P codes) for a well-baby exam, but all routine exams get a Z code! Codes for genetic carrier and genetic susceptibility to disease are covered in the second block, **Z14-Z15**.

The next five blocks have one code each, but all have indented codes under them and each one has notes. For example, Z16 *Resistance to antimicrobial drugs* has a **"Code first"** note and an **Excludes1** note.

Persons subject to potential health hazards related to communicable diseases are covered in **Block Z20-Z29**. This block also includes carrier of infectious disease and encounter for immunization.

Codes for health services to patients in circumstances related to reproduction are found in block **Z30-Z39**. They cover contraceptive management, procreative management and pregnancy.

Codes **Z40-Z53** are to be used to indicate a reason for care. These codes may be used for patients who already have been treated for a disease or injury and are receiving care following their treatment. Examples include plastic and reconstructive surgery following a medical procedure or healed injury, attention to artificial openings, fitting and adjustment of external prosthetic device, and care involving renal dialysis.

Codes **Z55-Z65** cover encounters related to socioeconomic and or psychosocial circumstances. For example, problems related to education and literacy, employment, unemployment, housing and other economic circumstances. Also, problems related to social environment, upbringing, and certain psychosocial circumstances.

Blocks **Z66 -Z68** are informational codes, such as do not resuscitate status, blood type, and body mass index (BMI). Codes Z69-Z76 cover health services in other circumstances such as mental health services related to abuse, and problems related to lifestyle.

The final block in this last chapter of the ICD-10 covers codes **Z77-Z99**, for contact with hazardous materials or substances, health status issues such as long-term drug therapy, family history of specified conditions, and personal history of specified conditions.

Let's work some exercises using the Z codes.

21.1

According to the Chapter-Specific Coding Guidelines, Z codes should always be used as:

_____ Principle diagnosis only
_____ Secondary diagnosis only
_____ Principle or secondary, depending on the circumstances

21.2

According to the Chapter-Specific Coding Guidelines, a status code and a history code are the same. True or False?

_____ True   _____ False

21.3

According to the Chapter-Specific Coding Guidelines, do screening and diagnostic examination mean the same thing?

_____ Yes, they are the same   _____ No, they are different

Take Note!
Is it a screening or diagnostic exam? Principal or secondary diagnosis? Status code or history code? It does make a difference. One of the most important jobs as a coder is to carefully read the Chapter-Specific Coding Guidelines. They can have a dramatic impact on coding.

21.1

A Z code can be used as either the <u>principle diagnosis or as a secondary diagnosis depending on the circumstances</u>.

However, certain Z codes can only be used as the principle diagnosis or first listed. For example, Z38 *Liveborn infants according to place of birth and type of delivery*. Certain other Z codes should only be listed as secondary (Z37 *Outcome of delivery*, for example). You will see a note informing you when one of these situations applies.

21.2

<u>False</u>. Status codes and history codes are not the same.

A status code indicates that a patient is either a carrier of a disease or has the residual of a past disease or condition. A history code indicates a past medical condition that no longer exists.

21.3

<u>No, they are different</u>.

A screening is an early detection test for disease in a patient who shows no signs of an illness. A diagnostic examination is done to rule out or confirm a suspected disease because the patient *does* have a sign or symptoms. The sign or symptom is used to explain the reason for the test.

QUICK QUIZ *Answers in Appendix A*

_____ 21.1	A condition resulting from another condition	*A.* Corrosions
_____ 21.2	Caused by chemicals	*B.* Burns
_____ 21.3	Caused by heat sources such as fire or hot appliances	*C.* Sequela
_____ 21.4	Injured tissue in which blood capillaries have been ruptured	*D.* Contusions

---

Use the Chapter-Specific Coding Guidelines to answer these questions.

21.4

Which of the following is true about observation codes?

_____ They are to be used only as the principle diagnosis code

_____ They are to be used only as a secondary diagnosis code

_____ They are used as principle diagnosis codes, but there is an exception

21.5

Can follow-up codes be used with history codes?

_____ Yes, follow-up codes can be used with history codes

_____ No, follow-up codes and history codes should not be used together

21.6

Should a Z code be used for a child's routine checkup?

_____ Yes, Z codes are used for routine child checkups

_____ No, child checkups are coded elsewhere

21.7

True or False? Nonspecific Z codes are designed to further clarify existing diagnoses and should be used with diagnosis codes from A00-T99.

_____ True   _____ False

There's a code for THAT??

Work with a pneumatic hammer and then feel like you're vibrating 24/7? Well, there's a code for that! T75.21 covers *Pneumatic hammer syndrome*.

21.4

Observation codes are used as the principle diagnosis codes, but there is an exception.

According to guideline *c. 6*, the only exception is when the principal diagnosis is required to be a code from category Z38.

21.5

Yes, follow-up codes can be used with history codes.

Follow-up codes are used to explain continued watching following completed treatment – that is, when the condition has been fully treated and no longer exists. Follow-up codes may be used with history codes to provide a full picture of the healed condition and its treatment. For a full explanation read follow-up *Section c. 8* in the Chapter-Specific Coding Guidelines.

21.6

Yes, the Z codes include codes for routine checkup.

Remember, all routine exams are Z codes.

21.7

False. Nonspecific Z codes are NOT designed to further clarify existing diagnoses and should NOT be used with most diagnosis codes from A00-T99.

Look again at the Chapter-Specific Coding Guidelines and find the section for nonspecific Z codes. There is little justification for using these codes with in-patients, and they should not be used in the outpatient setting except when the documentation does not provide more precise information. In other words, these codes should not be used very often.

21.8

You see a claim with both Z11.0 *Encounter for screening for intestinal infectious diseases* and Z00.00 *Encounter for general adult medical examination without abnormal findings*. Can these two codes be used at the same time?

_____ Yes, it is ok to use these codes at the same time
_____ No, these codes should not be used at the same time

21.9

Dr. Wellbeing conducts a routine examination of the patient's ears and finds nothing abnormal. It appears to you that Z01.10 is the appropriate code. Are you correct?

_____ Yes, Z01.10 is for the routine examination of ears without abnormal findings
_____ No, there is a note stating that Z01.10 should not be used for a routine examination

21.10

You see a chart with two codes: Z15.01 *Genetic susceptibility to malignant neoplasm of breast* and Z85.820 *Personal history of malignant melanoma of skin*. Should these two codes ever be used together?

_____ Yes, if applicable
_____ No, they should never be used together

21.11

You see a chart with codes C50.111 and Z17.0. Which is the proper order for these codes?

_____ C50.111 should be the principle diagnosis, followed by Z17.0
_____ Z17.0 should be the principle diagnosis, followed by C50.111
_____ It doesn't matter which is coded first

21.8

Yes, these codes can be used at the same time.

There is an **Excludes2** note after Z00 specifying that Z11-Z13 can be used with the Z00 codes.

21.9

Yes, Z01.10 is for the routine examination of ears without abnormal findings.

The note after Z01 states that these codes include the routine examination of a specific system. In this case the specific system is the ears.

21.10

Yes, there is a note saying they should be coded together if applicable.

How do you know? Because one of the notes after Z15.0 says to use additional codes, if applicable, for any personal history of malignant neoplasm (Z85.-).

21.11

C50.111 should be the principle diagnosis, followed by Z17.0.

Look up C50.11. You will see a **"Use additional code"** note under C50 regarding Z17.0 or Z17.1. This informs you to use Z17.0 or Z17.1 in addition to C50. Now look up Z17.0 There is a **"Code first"** note after Z17 that mentions C50.-. This means you must list the C50 code first.

QUICK QUIZ	*Answers in Appendix A*
_____ 21.5 Around or near	*A.* Retro
_____ 21.6 New	*B.* Peri
_____ 21.7 Behind	*C.* Neo
_____ 21.8 Prior to	*D.* Pre

21.12

Scan the Z codes. How many of them require a 7th character?

_____ One   _____ Four   _____ Twelve
_____ None of them   _____ All of them

21.13

You see a claim with code O28.3 followed by code Z36. Is this appropriate?

_____ Yes
_____ No

21.14

Samuel had an encounter for replacement of his complete artificial left arm prosthesis. Can this service be coded with one of the Z44 codes?

_____ Yes
_____ No

21.15

Which of these codes identifies a person who has the following blood type: Type AB blood, Rh negative

_____ Z67.3   _____ Z67.30
_____ Z67.31   _____ Z67.91

21.16

The patient is a genetic carrier of cystic fibrosis. Complete the code.

Z_____

21.12

The correct answer is <u>none of them</u>.

7th characters are not used with the Z codes.

21.13

The correct answer is <u>yes</u>.

Why? There is an **Excludes2** note that says they can be coded together. After code Z36 there is an **Excludes2** note covering all the O28 codes. So, codes O28.3 and Z36 can be used together.

21.14

The correct answer is <u>yes</u>.

Why? There is an **Includes** note indicating that removal or replacement of external prosthetic devices should be coded as Z44.

21.15

The answer is: <u>Z67.31</u> is the code for Type AB blood, Rh negative.

Z67.3 is the broad category for Type AB blood, but you always need to go to the most detailed level you can. Take a look:

Z67.30 is *Type AB blood, Rh positive* – but our patient is Rh negative

Z67.31 is *Type AB blood, Rh negative* – correct!

Z67.91 is *Unspecified blood type, Rh negative* – this code is for unspecified, but we know the blood type in this case is AB.

21.16

<u>Z14.1</u> is the correct code.

Looking at **Block Z14-Z15**, the second block, we see that Z14 is the code for *Genetic carrier* and Z14.1 further specifies *Cystic fibrosis carrier*. Always choose the most detailed code that applies.

Use the blocks at the beginning of the chapter to answer these questions.

21.17

John's screening report indicates that he has a retained foreign body fragment. It is made out of plastic. Complete the code.

Z_____

21.18

Mr. Jones' chart shows he has a body mass index (BMI) of 34.5. Complete the code.

Z_____

21.19

Paul has a resistance to antimicrobial drugs, specifically antiviral drugs. Complete the code.

Z_____

QUICK QUIZ *Answers in Appendix A*		
_____ 21.9 Stones	*A.*	-lysis
_____ 21.10 Movement	*B.*	Lith
_____ 21.11 Breaking down	*C.*	-kinesia
_____ 21.12 To pour out	*D.*	Effus(e)
_____ 21.13 Myo	*A.*	Joint
_____ 21.14 Myel	*B.*	Muscle
_____ 21.15 Dorso	*C.*	Back
_____ 21.16 Arthro	*D.*	spine

21.17

The correct code is Z18.2.

Go to the list of blocks at the beginning of the chapter and find the block for Retained foreign body fragment (**Z18**). Then, scan the indented list until you find retained plastic fragments.

21.18

Z68.34 is the correct code for an adult patient with a body mass index of 34.5.

Look at the list of blocks at the beginning of the chapter and find **Block Z68** (Body mass index (BMI)). Notice that the codes for adults are divided into groups of 19 or less, 20-29, 30-39 and 40 or greater. Code Z68.34 applies to a BMI of 34.5.

21.19

The correct code is Z16.33.

Start with Z16 *Resistance to antimicrobial drugs*. Look down the indented list to find *Resistance to antiviral drugs* and you will see code Z16.33.

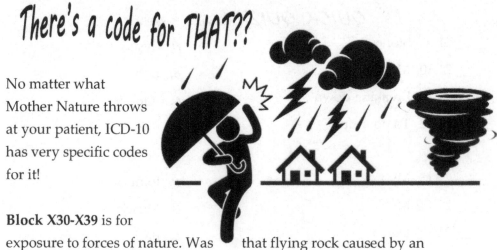

There's a code for THAT??

No matter what Mother Nature throws at your patient, ICD-10 has very specific codes for it!

Block X30-X39 is for exposure to forces of nature. Was that flying rock caused by an earthquake? Volcano? Tidal wave? Hurricane? Tornado? Some other cataclysmic storm? Make no mistake: it does matter whether the injury was due to an earthquake as opposed to a volcano!

Chapter Quiz (Answers in Appendix A)

Match the code to the block title the code is in.
NOTE: some blocks may be used more than once.

_____ 21.1 Z17.0	A. Persons encountering health services for examinations
_____ 21.2 Z45.02	B. Genetic carrier and genetic susceptibility to disease
_____ 21.3 Z62.0	C. Resistance to antimicrobial drugs
_____ 21.4 Z18.33	D. Estrogen receptor status
_____ 21.5 Z69.11	E. Retained foreign body fragments
_____ 21.6 Z85.830	F. Persons with potential health hazards related to communicable diseases
_____ 21.7 Z15.02	G. Persons encountering health services in circumstances related to reproduction
_____ 21.8 Z20.818	H. Encounters for other specific health care
_____ 21.9 Z66	I. Persons with potential health hazards related to socioeconomic and psychosocial circumstances
_____ 21.10 Z68.32	J. Do not resuscitate status
_____ 21.11 Z04.72	K. Blood type
_____ 21.12 Z74.01	L. Body mass index [BMI]
_____ 21.13 Z32.01	M. Persons encountering health services in other circumstances
_____ 21.14 Z16.24	N. Persons with potential health hazards related to family and personal history and certain conditions influencing health status
_____ 21.15 Z67	
_____ 21.16 Z12.11	

Indicate all appropriate notes for each code.

21.17 Z40.02 _____ _____ _____	A. **Includes**
21.18 Z47.1 _____ _____ _____	B. **Excludes1**
21.19 Z18.11 _____ _____	C. **Excludes2**
21.20 Z23 _____ _____	D. **"Use additional code"**
21.21 Z01.01 _____ _____ _____ _____	E. **"Code first"**
21.22 Z52.21 _____ _____ _____	F. **"Code also"**
21.23 Z3A.41 _____	
21.24 Z79.811 _____ _____ _____ _____ _____ _____	
21.25 Z16.21 _____ _____	
21.26 Z77.011 _____ _____ _____	
21.27 Z04.41 _____ _____	
21.28 Z45.2 _____ _____ _____	
21.29 Z31.83 _____ _____ _____	
21.30 Z87.51 _____ _____ _____ _____	
21.31 Z20.01 _____ _____	
21.32 Z71.1 _____ _____	
21.33 Z17.0 _____	
21.34 Z85.020 _____ _____ _____ _____	
21.35 Z51.11 _____ _____ _____	
21.36 Z15.01 _____ _____ _____ _____	
21.37 Z73.4 _____	

22

Codes for Special Purposes
Vaping-Related Disorder and Coronavirus Infections (COVID-19)

Chapter 22 of the ICD-10-CM was added for provisional assignment of new diseases of uncertain etiology or emergency use.

Currently there are three codes in this chapter:
> U07.0 *Vaping-related disorder*
> U07.1 *COVID-19*
> U09.9 *Post COVID-19 condition, unspecified*

Vaping-related disorders

Let's take a look at some of the guidelines for coding and reporting vaping-related disorders. You will find the vaping guidelines under Chapter 10 of the Coding Guidelines.

For patients presenting with condition(s) related to vaping, the principal diagnosis to assign is code U07.0, *Vaping-related disorder*. If vaping has caused a lung injury assign only code U07.0. Additional codes should be assigned for other manifestations. For example, assign codes from subcategory J96.0- for acute respiratory failure or use code J68.0 for pneumonitis.

Cough, shortness of breath and other associated respiratory signs and symptoms due to vaping should not be coded separately when a definitive diagnosis has been established. Gastrointestinal symptoms, such as diarrhea and abdominal pain should be coded separately.

COVID-19

Let's look at some of the guidelines for coding and reporting COVID-19 infections. Most of the COVID-19 guidelines are in the Chapter-Specific Coding Guidelines for Chapter 1 under Coronavirus infections.

a) Code only confirmed cases

The guidelines state that you should code only a confirmed diagnosis as documented by the provider, documentation of a positive COVID-19 test result, or a presumptive positive COVID-19 test result. Use code U07.1 *COVID-19* for a confirmed diagnosis.

Take Note! *Note that this is an exception to the hospital inpatient guideline Section II, H. In this context, "confirmation" does not require documentation of the type of test performed; the provider's documentation that the individual has COVID-19 is sufficient.*

Do not assign code U07.1 if the provider documents "suspected," "possible," "probable" or "inconclusive" COVID-19. Instead, assign a code(s) explaining the reason for the encounter (such as fever) or Z20.828, *Contact with and (suspected) exposure to other viral communicable diseases.*

b) Sequencing of codes

When COVID-19 is the principal diagnosis, code U07.1, *COVID-19,* should be the first code listed; it should be sequenced first. The appropriate codes for associated manifestations should follow. Note that there is an exception in the case of obstetrics, sepsis, or transplant complications.

A patient admitted or presenting for a health encounter because of COVID-19 during pregnancy, childbirth or the puerperium should receive a principal diagnosis code of O98.5-, *Other viral diseases complicating pregnancy, childbirth and the puerperium*. This should be followed by code U07.1 *COVID-19*, and the code(s) for any other manifestation(s). Codes from Chapter 15 should always be listed first.

c) Acute respiratory illness due to COVID-19

When the reason for the admission/encounter is a respiratory manifestation of COVID-19, assign code U07.1, *COVID-19* as the principal diagnosis and assign code(s) for the respiratory manifestation(s) as additional diagnoses.

(i) **Pneumonia**

For a pneumonia case that is confirmed due to COVID-19, use codes U07.1 *COVID-19* and J12.89 *Other viral pneumonia*.

(ii) **Acute bronchitis**

Assign codes U07.1 *COVID-19* and J20.8 *Acute bronchitis due to other specified organisms* when acute bronchitis is due to COVID-19. Bronchitis not otherwise specified (NOS) that is due to COVID-19 should be coded using codes U07.1 and J40 *Bronchitis, not specified as acute or chronic*.

(iii) **Lower respiratory infection**

If the COVID-19 is documented as being associated with a lower respiratory infection not otherwise specified (NOS), or an acute respiratory infection, NOS, use codes U07.1 and J22 *Unspecified acute lower respiratory infection*.

If the COVID-19 is documented as being associated with a respiratory infection NOS, use codes U07.1 and J98.8 *Other specified respiratory disorders*.

(iv) **Acute respiratory distress syndrome (ARDS)**

For a patient documented with acute respiratory distress syndrome due to COVID-19, use codes U07.1 and J80 *Acute respiratory distress syndrome*.

(v) **Acute respiratory failure**

For acute respiratory failure due to COVID-19, use code U07.1 and J96.0-.

d) Non-respiratory manifestations of COVID-19

For non-respiratory manifestations (e.g., viral enteritis) of COVID-19, use code U07.1 as the principal diagnosis and assign additional code(s) for manifestations.

e) Exposure to COVID-19

For asymptomatic people with actual or suspected exposure to COVID-19, and the exposed individual either tests negative or the test results are unknown, use code Z20.828 *Contact with and (suspected) exposure to other viral communicable diseases*. If the exposed individual tests positive for the COVID-19 virus, see **guideline a)**.

f) Screening for COVID-19

During the COVID-19 pandemic, a screening code is generally not appropriate. For COVID-19 testing, code as exposure to COVID-19 (**guideline e)**).

g) Signs and symptoms without definitive diagnosis of COVID-19

For patients presenting with any signs or symptoms that are associated with COVID-19 (such as fever, etc) but a definitive diagnosis has not been established, assign the appropriate code(s) for each of the presenting signs and symptoms such as: R05 *Cough,* R06.02 *Shortness of breath,* or R50.9 *Fever, unspecified*

If a patient with signs or symptoms associated with COVID-19 also has an actual or suspected contact with or exposure to COVID-19, assign code Z20.828 *Contact with and (suspected) exposure to other viral communicable diseases,* as an additional code.

h) Asymptomatic individuals who test positive for COVID-19

See **guideline a)** above for asymptomatic individuals who test positive for COVID-19. Although the individual is asymptomatic, they have tested positive and is considered to have the COVID-19 infection.

i) Personal history of COVID-19

Assign Z86.19, *Personal history of other infectious and parasitic diseases* for patients with a history of COVID-19.

j) Follow-up visits after COVID-19 infection has been resolved

For individuals who previously had COVID-19 and are being seen for follow-up evaluation and COVID-19 test results are negative, assign codes Z09, *Encounter for follow-up examination after completed treatment for conditions other than malignant neoplasm* and Z86.19, *Personal history of other infectious and parasitic diseases.*

k) Encounter for antibody testing

If the testing is not being performed to confirm a current COVID-19 infection, nor a follow-up test after resolution of COVID-19, assign Z01.84, *Encounter for antibody response examination,* otherwise follow the applicable guidelines above.

l) Multisystem Inflammatory Syndrome

If the patient has multisystem inflammatory syndrome (MIS) and COVID-19, assign code U07.1 as the principal diagnosis and assign code M35.81 as an additional diagnosis.

m) Post COVID-19 Condition

U09.9 is used for designating that the current condition is a post COVID-19 condition (associated symptoms or conditions that develop following a previous COVID-19 condition(s) related to the previous COVID-19 infection).

Let's work some practice exercises concerning the COVID-19 guidelines.

22.1

The current COVID-19 guidelines are the final guidelines.

_____ True   _____ False

22.2

Which code should be used for COVID-19?

_____ U07.0   _____ U07.1

22.3

Only confirmed cases of COVID-19 should be coded.

_____ True   _____ False

22.4

What is the correct sequencing of codes when COVID-19 is the principal diagnosis (excluding obstetrics, sepsis, or transplant patients)?

_____ Code U07.1 is listed first followed by U07.0
_____ Manifestations are listed first followed by U07.1
_____ U07.1 is listed first followed by only the primary manifestation
_____ U07.1 is listed first followed by all manifestations

22.1

The correct answer is <u>False</u>.

Chapter 22 is for *provisional* assignment of new diseases of uncertain etiology or emergency use. Because of the unprecedented nature of the pandemic, ICD-10-CM guidelines took effect April 1, 2020. Each year the ICD-10-CM is updated effective October 1 and the guidelines for COVID-19 may change in the next edition. The current guidelines are not necessarily the final guidelines.

22.2

The correct answer is <u>U07.1</u>.

U07.1 is the code for COVID-19. U07.0 is used for Vaping-related disorder.

22.3

The correct answer is <u>True</u>.

Only confirmed cases of COVID-19 should be coded. Confirmation does not require documentation of a positive test result for COVID-19. The provider's documentation that the patient has COVID-19 is sufficient.

22.4

The correct answer is <u>U07.1 is listed first followed by all manifestations</u>.

When COVID-19 is the principal diagnosis, code U07.1, *COVID-19*, should be the first code listed, it should be sequenced first. The appropriate codes for associated manifestations should follow. Remember, there is an exception for obstetric, sepsis, or transplant patients. For example, obstetric patients should have a principal diagnosis code of O98.5-, *Other viral diseases complicating pregnancy, childbirth and the puerperium*. This should be followed by U07.1 for COVID-19.

22.5

Which code combination should you use for a patient with COVID-19 and acute bronchitis?

_____ U07.1 and J80   _____ U07.1 and J40

_____ U07.1 and J20.8   _____ U07.1 and J22

_____ U07.1 and J98.8   _____ U07.1 and J12.89

22.6

Which code combination should you use for a patient with COVID-19 and pneumonia?

_____ U07.1 and J80   _____ U07.1 and J40

_____ U07.1 and J20.8   _____ U07.1 and J22

_____ U07.1 and J98.8   _____ U07.1 and J12.89

22.7

Which code combination should you use for a patient with COVID-19 and lower respiratory infection, not otherwise specified (NOS)?

_____ U07.1 and J80   _____ U07.1 and J40

_____ U07.1 and J20.8   _____ U07.1 and J22

_____ U07.1 and J98.8   _____ U07.1 and J12.89

22.8

Which code combination should you use for a patient with COVID-19 and acute respiratory distress syndrome (ARDS)?

_____ U07.1 and J80   _____ U07.1 and J40

_____ U07.1 and J20.8   _____ U07.1 and J22

_____ U07.1 and J98.8   _____ U07.1 and J12.89

22.5

The correct answer is <u>U07.1 and J20.8</u>.

Assign codes U07.1 *COVID-19* and J20.8 *Acute bronchitis due to other specified organisms* when acute bronchitis is due to COVID-19.

22.6

The correct answer is <u>U07.1 and J12.89.</u>

For a pneumonia case that is confirmed due to COVID-19, use codes U07.1 *COVID-19* and J12.89 *Other viral pneumonia*.

22.7

The correct answer is <u>U07.1 and J22</u>.

If the COVID-19 is documented as being associated with a lower respiratory infection not otherwise specified (NOS), or an acute respiratory infection, NOS, use codes U07.1 and J22 *Unspecified acute lower respiratory infection*.

22.8

The correct answer is <u>U07.1 and J80</u>.

For a patient documented with acute respiratory distress syndrome due to COVID-19, use codes U07.1 and J80 *Acute respiratory distress syndrome*.

QUICK QUIZ *Answers in Appendix A*	
_____ 22.1 Acute bronchitis	*A.* J22
_____ 22.2 Acute respiratory infection, NOS	*B.* J96.0-
_____ 22.3 COVID-19	*C.* J20.8
_____ 22.4 Acute respiratory failure	*D.* U07.1

22.9

Which code combination should you use for a patient with COVID-19 and bronchitis not otherwise specified (NOS)?

_____ U07.1 and J80	_____ U07.1 and J40
_____ U07.1 and J20.8	_____ U07.1 and J22
_____ U07.1 and J98.8	_____ U07.1 and J12.89

22.10

Which code combination should you use for a patient with COVID-19 and respiratory infection not otherwise specified (NOS)?

_____ U07.1 and J80	_____ U07.1 and J40
_____ U07.1 and J20.8	_____ U07.1 and J22
_____ U07.1 and J98.8	_____ U07.1 and J12.89

22.11

For individuals with a personal history of COVID-19, which code(s) should you assign?

_____ U07.1	_____ Z09 and Z86.19
_____ Z86.19	_____ Z20.828

22.12

When a patient has an encounter for antibody testing and the testing is not being performed to confirm a current COVID-19 infection, nor a follow-up test after resolution of COVID-19, which code should you assign?

_____ U07.1	_____ Z20.828
_____ Z11.59	_____ Z01.84

22.13

True or False? Do not assign codes for non-respiratory manifestations of COVID-19.

_____ True	_____ False

22.9

The correct answer is <u>U07.1 and J40</u>.

Bronchitis not otherwise specified (NOS) that is due to COVID-19 should be coded using codes U07.1 and J40 *Bronchitis, not specified as acute or chronic*.

22.10

The correct answer is <u>U07.1 and J98.8</u>.

If COVID-19 is documented as being associated with a respiratory infection NOS, use codes U07.1 and J98.8 *Other specified respiratory disorders*.

22.11

The correct answer is <u>Z86.19</u>.

For patients with a personal history of COVID-19, assign Z86.19 *Personal history of other infectious and parasitic diseases*.

22.12

The correct answer is <u>Z01.84</u>.

When a patient has an encounter for antibody testing and the testing is not being performed to confirm a current COVID-19 infection, nor a follow-up test after resolution of COVID-19, assign code Z01.84 *Encounter for antibody response examination*.

22.13

The correct answer is <u>False</u>.

When the reason for the encounter or admission is a non-respiratory manifestation (for example, viral enteritis) of COVID-19, assign code U07.1 as the principal diagnosis and assign the code(s) for the manifestation(s) as additional diagnoses.

22.14

For asymptomatic individuals where there is an actual exposure to someone who is confirmed or suspected to have COVD-19, and the exposed individual either tests negative or the test results are unknown, which code should you assign?

_____ U07.1   _____ Z20.828

_____ Z11.59   _____ Z03.818

22.15

If an asymptomatic person is screened for COVID-19 and tests positive, which code should you assign?

_____ U07.1   _____ Z20.828

_____ Z11.59   _____ Z03.818

22.16

For patients presenting with signs or symptoms associated with COVID-19 but a definitive diagnosis has not been established, how do you assign the codes?

_____ Assign code U07.1

_____ Assign the appropriate code(s) for each of the presenting signs and
         symptoms

_____ Assign code U07.1 and also assign the appropriate code(s) for each of the
         presenting signs and symptoms

22.17

If the provider documents "suspected" or "probable" COVID-19 what is the proper way to code this?

_____ U07.1

_____ Code the signs and symptoms reported

_____ U07.1 first, then the signs and symptoms reported

_____ U07.0

22.14

The correct answer is <u>Z20.828</u>.

When there is an actual exposure to someone who is confirmed or suspected (not ruled out) to have COVID-19, and the exposed individual either tests negative or the test results are unknown, use code Z20.828 *Contact with and (suspected) exposure to other viral communicable diseases*. If the exposed individual tests positive for the COVID-19 virus, see **guideline a)** at the beginning of this chapter.

22.15

The correct answer is <u>U07.1</u>.

If an asymptomatic person is screened for COVID-19 and tests positive use code U07.1. See **guideline a)** at the beginning of this chapter.

22.16

The correct answer is <u>Assign the appropriate code(s) for each of the presenting signs and symptoms</u>.

For patients presenting with any signs or symptoms that are associated with COVID-19 (such as fever, etc) but a definitive diagnosis has not been established, assign the appropriate code(s) for each of the presenting signs and symptoms such as:

R05 *Cough*

R06.02 *Shortness of breath*

R50.9 *Fever, unspecified*

22.17

The correct answer is <u>Code the signs and symptoms reported</u>.

Code U07.1 is for confirmed cases only. For "suspected," "possible," "probable" or "inconclusive" COVID-19 you should assign a code(s) explaining the reason for the encounter, that is, the signs and symptoms reported.

Chapter Quiz (Answers in Appendix A)

Choose the correct code(s) for each scenario.

_____ 22.1	The provider documents acute respiratory failure due to COVID-19.	A. U07.1 and J98.8
_____ 22.2	The patient has acute bronchitis confirmed due to COVID-19.	B. U07.1 and J22
_____ 22.3	The COVID-19 is documented as being associated with a respiratory infection, NOS.	C. U07.1 and J96.0-
_____ 22.4	An individual with a personal history of COVID-19.	D. U09.9
_____ 22.5	The COVID-19 is documented as being associated with a lower respiratory infection, not otherwise specified (NOS)	E. U07.1 and J20.8
_____ 22.6	A patient has an encounter for antibody testing. The testing is not being performed to confirm a current COVID-19 infection, nor a follow-up test after resolution of COVID-19.	F. R05
_____ 22.7	The patient has a cough but a definitive diagnosis of COVID-19 has not been established.	G. U07.1 and J80
_____ 22.8	The patient has bronchitis not otherwise specified (NOS) which is due to COVID-19.	H. Z86.19
_____ 22.9	The patient had COVID-19 previously and is now presenting with a condition related to COVID-19.	I. Z01.84
_____ 22.10	The patient has acute respiratory distress syndrome (ARDS) due to COVID-19.	J. U07.1 and J40

Chapter Quiz (Answers in Appendix A)

Choose the correct code(s) for each scenario.
NOTE: some codes may be used more than once.

_____ 22.11 During pregnancy a patient presents for a health care encounter and she tests positive for COVID-19.	A. U07.1
_____ 22.12 A patient with signs/symptoms associated with COVID-19 who also has an actual contact with someone who has COVID-19.	B. U07.1 and J22
_____ 22.13 There was an actual exposure to someone who is confirmed to have COVID-19 and the exposed individual tests negative.	C. O98.5- and U07.1
_____ 22.14 The patient presents with shortness of breath but has not been tested for COVID-19.	D. R50.9
_____ 22.15 An asymptomatic patient tests positive for COVID-19.	E. Z20.828
_____ 22.16 The patient presents with fever, unspecified but no diagnosis of COVID-19 has been established.	F. U07.1 and Z20.828
_____ 22.17 A patient with no known exposure to the virus but with a confirmed diagnosis of COVID-19.	G. R06.02
_____ 22.18 The provider documents "inconclusive" COVID-19.	H. Only code symptoms
_____ 22.19 A patient with COVID-19 documented as being associated with an acute respiratory infection, NOS.	
_____ 22.20 A patient admitted for childbirth who has COVID-19.	

Final Review

Congratulations! You've made it to the finish line. Take a moment to relax and pat yourself on the back. Hopefully you will not be suffering from R41.0, H53.2, F43.0 or R57. When you're ready, forge ahead to these wrap-up exercises. Working through them, you'll be surprised at the extensive knowledge you've gained.

You should now be very comfortable with the massive new 70,000+ code ICD-10-CM book and how it is organized. You've practiced **hands-on coding,** and **built skills** that are critical to winning a **top paying job** in the health care billing and reimbursement fields. You've picked up scores of **inside tips** that in many cases can even **put you ahead** of coders with years of practice!

By gaining an understanding of many of the most common **Greek and Latin** word parts, you also are able to figure out many multi-syllable medical terms you have never seen before.

While you may currently, or at some point in your career, work in a specialized practice and concentrate on only a few of the chapters, the **broad knowledge** you have gained here can put you **ahead of the game** as you encounter new or **expanded career opportunities**.

The following pages give you one final chance to showcase your amazing new skills. Best of luck to you as you use them to further your career!

...RAS

Final Review (Answers in Appendix A)

Fill in the first letter of codes in each chapter. NOTE: use H twice.

_____ 1.	Respiratory System	A. Codes begin with A or B
_____ 2.	Symptoms and Signs	C. Codes begin with C or D
_____ 3.	Ear and Mastoid Process	D. Codes begin with D
_____ 4.	Endocrine Diseases	E. Codes begin with E
_____ 5.	Musculoskeletal System	F. Codes begin with F
_____ 6.	Nervous System	G. Codes begin with G
_____ 7.	Genitourinary System	H. Codes begin with H
_____ 8.	Mental and Behavioral	H. Codes begin with H
_____ 9.	Injuries or Poisoning	I. Codes begin with I
_____ 10.	Neoplasms	J. Codes begin with J
_____ 11.	Digestive System	K. Codes begin with K
_____ 12.	Certain Infectious Diseases	L. Codes begin with L
_____ 13.	Diseases of the Blood	M. Codes begin with M
_____ 14.	Skin and Subcutaneous Tissue	N. Codes begin with N
_____ 15.	The Perinatal Period	O. Codes begin with O
_____ 16.	Factors Influencing Health	P. Codes begin with P
_____ 17.	Pregnancy	Q. Codes begin with Q
_____ 18.	Circulatory System	R. Codes begin with R
_____ 19.	Congenital Malformations	S. Codes begin with S or T
_____ 20.	Eye and Adnexa	Z. Codes begin with Z

Match the definition to the term.

_____ 21.	Producing a fever	A. Osteomalacia
_____ 22.	Enlargement of a body part	B. Cholelithiasis
_____ 23.	Softening of the bones	C. Glossodynia
_____ 24.	Refers to the outermost layer of skin	D. Spondylolysis
_____ 25.	Difficult movement of an organ	E. Epidermal
_____ 26.	Abnormal flow of blood	F. Lymphadenitis
_____ 27.	Below the skin	G. Pyrogenic
_____ 28.	Abnormal development of an organ	H. Hypertrophy
_____ 29.	Stones in the gallbladder	I. Arthropathy
_____ 30.	Painful tongue	J. Tachypnea
_____ 31.	Temporary deficiency of blood in a body part	K. Ischemia
		L. Osteomyelitis
_____ 32.	Inflamed lymph nodes	M. Glossitis
_____ 33.	Stiff joints	N. Subcutaneous
_____ 34.	Breaking down of a vertebral structure	O. Dysplasia
_____ 35.	Disease of the joint	P. Nephrogenic
_____ 36.	Rapid breathing	Q. Hemorrhage
_____ 37.	Bleeding into the joints	R. Dyskinesia
_____ 38.	Inflammation of bone and bone marrow	S. Hemarthrosis
_____ 39.	Arising from the kidney	T. Ankylosis
_____ 40.	Inflammation of the tongue	

Match the code to the description.

_____ 41.	L23.81	A.	Encounter for full-term uncomplicated delivery
_____ 42.	P70.2	B.	Swimmer's ear, bilateral
_____ 43.	V43.64	C.	Interstitial cystitis (chronic) without hematuria
_____ 44.	S51.032A	D.	Overdose of radiation given during therapy
_____ 45.	Q30.0	E.	Autosomal recessive ocular albinism
_____ 46.	R31.21	F.	Retained magnetic metal fragments
_____ 47.	E70.311	G.	Acute appendicitis with localized peritonitis
_____ 48.	T33.42	H.	Pneumonia due to Escherichia coli
_____ 49.	M86.052	I.	Exposure to excessive natural heat, initial encounter
_____ 50.	Z18.11	J.	Neonatal diabetes mellitus
_____ 51.	I08.3	K.	Puncture wound without foreign body of left elbow, initial encounter
_____ 52.	N30.10	L.	Episodic cluster headache, intractable
_____ 53.	G44.011	M.	Allergic contact dermatitis due to animal dander
_____ 54.	W20.0XXS	N.	Car passenger injured in collision with van in traffic accident
_____ 55.	K35.30	O.	Combined rheumatic disorders of mitral, aortic and tricuspid valves
_____ 56.	J15.5	P.	Asymptomatic microscopic hematuria
_____ 57.	X30.XXXA	Q.	Choanal atresia
_____ 58.	Y63.2	R.	Superficial frostbite of left arm
_____ 59.	O80	S.	Struck by falling object in cave-in, sequala
_____ 60.	H60.333	T.	Acute hematogenous osteomyelitis, left femur

Use the alphabetical index to find the code for each description.

_____ 61. Angina pectoris with documented spasm

_____ 62. Thyrotoxicosis with diffuse goiter with thyrotoxic crisis or storm

_____ 63. Allergic contact dermatitis due to drugs in contact with skin

_____ 64. Acute bronchitis due to streptococcus

_____ 65. Infective myositis, right ankle

_____ 66. Central retinal vein occlusion, left eye, with macular edema

_____ 67. Abnormal blood level of cobalt

_____ 68. Acute hepatitis C with hepatic coma

_____ 69. Polyhydramnios, second trimester, single gestation

_____ 70. Chronic obstructive pyelonephritis

_____ 71. Acquired stenosis of left external ear canal secondary to inflammation and infection

_____ 72. Cutaneous listeriosis

_____ 73. Contusion of left great toe without damage to nail, subsequent encounter

_____ 74. Acute appendicitis with localized peritonitis

_____ 75. Fear of injections and transfusions

_____ 76. Burn of first degree of chin, initial encounter

_____ 77. Congenital aneurysm of aorta

_____ 78. Transitory neonatal hyperthyroidism

_____ 79. Iron deficiency anemia secondary to blood loss (chronic)

_____ 80. Generalized idiopathic epilepsy and epileptic syndromes, intractable, without status epilepticus

Match the description to the note.

_____ 81. The codes should never be used at the same time

_____ 82. Example of content in a category

_____ 83. You must use a different code, but can be used at the same time

_____ 84. The underlying condition should be coded first

_____ 85. Another code should be used, but does not specify which code should be first

A. **Includes**

B. **Excludes1**

C. **Excludes2**

D. **"Code also"**

E. Etiology/manifestation

Indicate all appropriate notes for each code.

86. O34.02 _____ _____ _____ _____ _____

87. S60.022 _____ _____ _____ _____

88. N60.12 _____ _____ _____

89. V43.01 _____ _____ _____ _____ _____

90. L64.0 _____ _____ _____ _____

91. R50.81 _____ _____ _____

92. Z00.110 _____ _____ _____

93. M60.212 _____ _____ _____

94. Q05.3 _____ _____ _____ _____

95. K22.10 _____ _____ _____ _____

96. X36.1 _____ _____ _____ _____

97. P83.30 _____ _____ _____

98. T20.112 _____ _____ _____ _____ _____

A. **Includes**

B. **Excludes1**

C. **Excludes2**

D. **"Use additional code"**

E. **"Code first"**

F. **"7th character"**

Appendix A

The following pages provide all the answers to the Quick Quizzes, Chapter Quizzes, Half-time Review and Final Review.

There's a code for THAT??

Who knew? Going even one night without sleep causes as much impairment as being legally intoxicated. It's called sleep deprivation, code Z72.820. Insomnia is different. See code G47.0-.

Basic Concepts
Quick Quiz:

1.   B.
2.   D.
3.   A.
4.   C.
5.   D.
6.   A.
7.   C.
8.   B.

Chapter 1
Chapter Quiz

1.1   D.
1.2   G.
1.3   K.
1.4   I.
1.5   N.
1.6   L.
1.7   J.
1.8   A.
1.9   R.
1.10 F.
1.11 Q.
1.12 H.
1.13 M.
1.14 B.
1.15 T.
1.16 E.
1.17 P.
1.18 S.
1.19 O.
1.20 C.
1.21 S.
1.22 L.
1.23 J.
1.24 Z.
1.25 I.
1.26 A.
1.27 P.

1.28 F.
1.29 D.
1.30 K.
1.31 M.
1.32 E.
1.33 R.
1.34 N.
1.35 H.
1.36 G.
1.37 C.
1.38 Q.
1.39 H.
1.40 O.

Chapter 2
Quick Quiz:

2.1   B.
2.2   C.
2.3   D.
2.4   A.
2.5   B.
2.6   D.
2.7   C.
2.8   A.
2.9   A.
2.10 C.
2.11 B.
2.12 D.
2.13 B.
2.14 D.
2.15 A.
2.16 C.

Chapter 2
Chapter Quiz

2.1   E.
2.2   J.
2.3   A.
2.4   F.
2.5   B.

2.6   G.
2.7   H.
2.8   C.
2.9   D.
2.10 I.
2.11 H.
2.12 F.
2.13 I.
2.14 G.
2.15 A.
2.16 D.
2.17 C.
2.18 B.
2.19 J.
2.20 E.
2.21 K.
2.22 Q.
2.23 N.
2.24 I.
2.25 M.
2.26 T.
2.27 O.
2.28 R.
2.29 D.
2.30 L.
2.31 A.
2.32 J.
2.33 E.
2.34 C.
2.35 G.
2.36 S.
2.37 B.
2.38 H.
2.39 P.
2.40 F.

Chapter 3
Quick Quiz:

3.1   D.
3.2   C.
3.3   B.

3.4 A.
3.5 B.
3.6 C.
3.7 D.
3.8 A.
3.9 C.
3.10 B.
3.11 D.
3.12 A.

Chapter 3
Chapter Quiz

3.1 A.
3.2 I.
3.3 L.
3.4 M.
3.5 B.
3.6 H.
3.7 E.
3.8 D.
3.9 F.
3.10 G.
3.11 C.
3.12 K.
3.13 J.
3.14 C.
3.15 F.
3.16 A.
3.17 D.
3.18 G.
3.19 B.
3.20 E.
3.21 E.
3.22 B.
3.23 A.
3.24 C.
3.25 G.
3.26 F.
3.27 H.
3.28 D.
3.29 K

3.30 D
3.31 E
3.32 L
3.33 Q
3.34 Z
3.35 H
3.36 I
3.37 G
3.38 V, W, X, Y
3.39 R
3.40 C, D

Chapter 4
Quick Quiz:

4.1 C.
4.2 B.
4.3 A.
4.4 D.
4.5 C.
4.6 A.
4.7 D.
4.8 B.

Chapter 4
Chapter Quiz

4.1 F.
4.2 H.
4.3 I. or L.
4.4 A.
4.5 Q.
4.6 B.
4.7 K.
4.8 R.
4.9 C.
4.10 P.
4.11 E.
4.12 G.
4.13 N.
4.14 S.
4.15 L. or I.

4.16 O.
4.17 M.
4.18 T.
4.19 D.
4.20 J.
4.21 C.
4.22 B.
4.23 F.
4.24 J.
4.25 A.
4.26 D.
4.27 G.
4.28 E.
4.29 H.
4.30 I.
4.31 H.
4.32 I.
4.33 G.
4.34 B.
4.35 E
4.36 A.
4.37 F.
4.38 J.
4.39 D.
4.40 C.

Chapter 5
Quick Quiz:

5.1 A.
5.2 D.
5.3 C.
5.4 B.
5.5 C.
5.6 B.
5.7 D.
5.8 A.

Chapter 5
Chapter Quiz

5.1   H.
5.2   E.
5.3   G.
5.4   F.
5.5   D.
5.6   B.
5.7   C.
5.8   A.
5.9   J.
5.10 A.
5.11 F.
5.12 K.
5.13 H.
5.14 L.
5.15 E.
5.16 G.
5.17 B.
5.18 C.
5.19 D.
5.20 I.
5.21 D.
5.22 H.
5.23 F.
5.24 K.
5.25 A.
5.26 G.
5.27 C.
5.28 E.
5.29 I.
5.30 B.
5.31 J.
5.32 A. C.
5.33 A. B. C.
5.34 A. B. C. D.
5.35 A. C.
5.36 A. B. C. E.
5.37 A. B. C.
5.38 A. B. C.

Chapter 6
Quick Quiz:

6.1   B.
6.2   A.
6.3   C.
6.4   D.

Chapter 6
Chapter Quiz

6.1   M.
6.2   H.
6.3   G.
6.4   L.
6.5   N.
6.6   I.
6.7   C.
6.8   A.
6.9   E.
6.10 B.
6.11 P.
6.12 J.
6.13 F.
6.14 D.
6.15 K.
6.16 O.
6.17 G25.61
6.18 G40.822
6.19 G37.4
6.20 G91.1
6.21 G04.02
6.22 G62.82
6.23 G81.01
6.24 G11.4
6.25 G71.0
6.26 G57.01
6.27 G31.2
6.28 P
6.29 Z
6.30 C or D
6.31 H

6.32 N
6.33 A or B
6.34 E
6.35 F
6.36 L

Chapter 7
Quick Quiz:

7.1   B.
7.2   A.
7.3   D.
7.4   C.
7.5   C.
7.6   D.
7.7   A.
7.8   B.
7.9   B.
7.10 D.
7.11 C.
7.12 A.

Chapter 7
Chapter Quiz

7.1   F.
7.2   E.
7.3   D.
7.4   A.
7.5   B.
7.6   C.
7.7   No
7.8   Yes
7.9   No
7.10 Yes
7.11 No
7.12 Yes
7.13 Yes
7.14 Yes
7.15 No
7.16 No
7.17 Yes

7.18	No
7.19	1
7.20	1
7.21	1
7.22	1
7.23	No
7.24	0
7.25	No
7.26	1
7.27	1
7.28	0
7.29	0
7.30	0
7.31	C.
7.32	D.
7.33	H.
7.34	F.
7.35	J.
7.36	L.
7.37	B.
7.38	A.
7.39	G.
7.40	K.
7.41	E.
7.42	I.
7.43	H
7.44	C or D
7.45	F
7.46	G
7.47	D
7.48	A or B
7.49	K
7.50	E

Chapter 8
Quick Quiz:

8.1	D.
8.2	A.
8.3	B.
8.4	C.
8.5	B.
8.6	D.
8.7	A.
8.8	C.
8.9	C.
8.10	A.
8.11	D.
8.12	B.
8.13	A.
8.14	B.
8.15	C.
8.16	D.
8.17	B.
8.18	D.
8.19	A.
8.20	C.

Chapter 8
Chapter Quiz

8.1	F.
8.2	A.
8.3	G.
8.4	D.
8.5	B.
8.6	C.
8.7	E.
8.8	D.
8.9	C.
8.10	C.
8.11	B.
8.12	C.
8.13	B.
8.14	A.
8.15	B.
8.16	C.
8.17	B.
8.18	D.
8.19	B.
8.20	A.
8.21	C.
8.22	A.
8.23	B.
8.24	C.
8.25	A.
8.26	D.
8.27	B.
8.28	C.
8.29	A.
8.30	B.
8.31	B.
8.32	D.
8.33	B.
8.34	C.
8.35	D.
8.36	B.
8.37	D.
8.38	E.
8.39	D.
8.40	A.

Chapter 9
Quick Quiz:

9.1	D.
9.2	C.
9.3	A.
9.4	B.
9.5	A.
9.6	C.
9.7	B.
9.8	D.

Chapter 9
Chapter Quiz

9.1	G.
9.2	H.
9.3	M.
9.4	I.
9.5	P.
9.6	L.
9.7	K.
9.8	C.
9.9	O.

9.10 B.	10.11 B.	**HALF-TIME**
9.11 D.	10.12 C.	**REVIEW**
9.12 A.		1. F.
9.13 F.	**Chapter 10**	2. N.
9.14 E.	**Chapter Quiz**	3. J.
9.15 Q.	10.1 C.	4. G.
9.16 N.	10.2 F.	5. M.
9.17 J.	10.3 A.	6. D.
9.18 I95.2	10.4 E.	7. O.
9.19 I30.0	10.5 D.	8. P.
9.20 I25.83	10.6 B.	9. L.
9.21 I69.090	10.7 intermittent	10. A.
9.22 I01.1	10.8 acute	11. K.
9.23 I10	10.9 chronic	12. B.
9.24 I42.1	10.10 acute	13. C.
9.25 I80.292	10.11 chronic	14. I.
9.26 I60.01	10.12 persistent	15. E.
9.27 I26.02	10.13 acute	16. H.
9.28 C. D.	10.14 chronic	17. I.
9.29 B. C. D.	10.15 acute	18. K.
9.30 B. C. D.	10.16 acute	19. F.
9.31 A. C. E.	10.17 chronic	20. Z.
9.32 A. B. C. D.	10.18 F.	21. H.
9.33 A. C. D.	10.19 C.	22. R.
9.34 C. D. E.	10.20 J.	23. C.
9.35 B. C. E.	10.21 E.	24. J.
9.36 A. B. C. E.	10.22 A.	25. G.
	10.23 K.	26. L.
Chapter 10	10.24 G.	27. O.
Quick Quiz:	10.25 I.	28. Q.
10.1 A.	10.26 H.	29. A.
10.2 B.	10.27 D.	30. H.
10.3 D.	10.28 B.	31. S.
10.4 C.	10.29 B. C. D.	32. D.
10.5 D.	10.30 A. B. C. D.	33. P.
10.6 A.	10.31 A. B. C. D.	34. E.
10.7 C.	10.32 B. C. D. E.	35. N.
10.8 B.	10.33 A. B. C. D.	36. M.
10.9 A.	10.34 B. C. D.	37. R.
10.10 D.	10.35 A. C. D.	38. M.
	10.36 B. C. D. E.	39. J.

40. H.
41. K.
42. P.
43. Q.
44. B.
45. N.
46. A.
47. O.
48. E.
49. F.
50. C.
51. S.
52. D.
53. I.
54. T.
55. L.
56. G.
57. I.
58. N.
59. O.
60. P.
61. C.
62. K.
63. B.
64. G.
65. D.
66. A.
67. F.
68. J.
69. M.
70. L.
71. E.
72. H.
73. D.
74. E.
75. A.
76. C.
77. B.
78. B. C.
79. B. C. E.
80. A. C. D.

81. A. B. C. D.
82. A. B. C. D.
83. B. C. E.
84. B. D. E.
85. B. C. D.
86. A. B. C.
87. B. C.
88. A. B. C. D.
89. B. C.
90. B. C. E.

Chapter 11
Quick Quiz:
11.1 B.
11.2 D.
11.3 A.
11.4 C.
11.5 C.
11.6 A.
11.7 B.
11.8 D.

Chapter 11
Chapter Quiz
11.1 P.
11.2 J.
11.3 H.
11.4 G.
11.5 A.
11.6 E.
11.7 M.
11.8 S.
11.9 D.
11.10 C.
11.11 N.
11.12 Q.
11.13 R.
11.14 F.
11.15 T.
11.16 I.

11.17 B.
11.18 O.
11.19 L.
11.20 K.
11.21 D.
11.22 E.
11.23 F.
11.24 H.
11.25 G.
11.26 J.
11.27 I.
11.28 A.
11.29 C.
11.30 B.
11.31 D.
11.32 C.
11.33 G.
11.34 J.
11.35 B.
11.36 F.
11.37 H.
11.38 E.
11.39 I.
11.40 A.

Chapter 12
Quick Quiz:
12.1 B.
12.2 D.
12.3 C.
12.4 A.
12.5 C.
12.6 A.
12.7 D.
12.8 B.

Chapter 12
Chapter Quiz
12.1 A.
12.2 C.

12.3 B.
12.4 E.
12.5 D.
12.6 I
12.7 F.
12.8 L.
12.9 A.
12.10 J.
12.11 G.
12.12 E.
12.13 D.
12.14 C.
12.15 H.
12.16 B.
12.17 M.
12.18 K.
12.19 L12.30
12.20 L41.3
12.21 L58.0
12.22 L89.624
12.23 L02.821
12.24 L24.2
12.25 L71.8
12.26 L50.0
12.27 L66.4
12.28 B. C. D.
12.29 B. C.
12.30 C. D.
12.31 C. D.
12.32 B. C. D.
12.33 A. C.
12.34 B. C.
12.35 A. B. C. D.
12.36 B. C. E.
12.37 B. C. D.
12.38 B. C. D.

Chapter 13
Chapter Quiz
13.1 K.
13.2 H.

13.3 O.
13.4 A.
13.5 L.
13.6 M.
13.7 Q.
13.8 E.
13.9 N.
13.10 T.
13.11 C.
13.12 P.
13.13 S.
13.14 F.
13.15 R.
13.16 D.
13.17 J.
13.18 G.
13.19 I.
13.20 B.
13.21 G.
13.22 P.
13.23 J.
13.24 F.
13.25 T.
13.26 I.
13.27 N.
13.28 E.
13.29 M.
13.30 K.
13.31 C.
13.32 H.
13.33 Q.
13.34 D.
13.35 O.
13.36 L.
13.37 A.
13.38 R.
13.39 B.
13.40 S.

Chapter 14
Quick Quiz:
14.1 A.
14.2 B.
14.3 D.
14.4 C.
14.5 C.
14.6 A.
14.7 D.
14.8 B.

Chapter 14
Chapter Quiz
14.1 C.
14.2 K.
14.3 H.
14.4 B.
14.5 I.
14.6 J.
14.7 A.
14.8 M.
14.9 L.
14.10 D.
14.11 N.
14.12 G.
14.13 E.
14.14 F.
14.15 A.
14.16 A.
14.17 A.
14.18 B.
14.19 A.
14.20 B.
14.21 D.
14.22 H.
14.23 G.
14.24 B.
14.25 J.
14.26 E.
14.27 I.

14.28 F.
14.29 A.
14.30 C.
14.31 K.
14.32 B. C. F.
14.33 C. D.
14.34 B. C. E.
14.35 B. C.
14.36 A. B. C. F.
14.37 B. C. D.
14.38 A. B. C. D.
14.39 B. C.

Chapter 15
Chapter Quiz
15.1 C.
15.2 F.
15.3 E.
15.4 A.
15.5 B.
15.6 D.
15.7 E
15.8 O
15.9 P
15.10 G
15.11 K
15.12 H
15.13 C or D
15.14 J
15.15 I
15.16 F
15.17 L
15.18 M
15.19 N
15.20 A or B
15.21 D.
15.22 F.
15.23 B.
15.24 C.
15.25 I.
15.26 A.

15.27 E.
15.28 G.
15.29 H.
15.30 A. B. C. D.
15.31 A. B. C. D. G.
15.32 B. C. D.
15.33 B. C. D. F.
15.34 A. B. C. D.
15.35 A. B. C. D. E.
15.36 A. B. C. D. G.
15.37 A. B. C. D. F. G.
15.38 B. C. D.
15.39 B. C. D. F.

Chapter 16
Quick Quiz:
16.1 B.
16.2 C.
16.3 D.
16.4 A.

Chapter 16
Chapter Quiz
16.1 C or D
16.2 F
16.3 I
16.4 O
16.5 K
16.6 Q
16.7 A or B
16.8 M
16.9 S or T
16.10 D
16.11 G
16.12 P
16.13 E
16.14 J
16.15 N
16.16 H
16.17 L

16.18 R
16.19 A. B. C. D.
16.20 A. B. C. E.
16.21 A. C.
16.22 A. B. C. D. E.
16.23 A. C. E.
16.24 A. B. C.
16.25 A. C.
16.26 A. C. E.
16.27 A. B. C. D.
16.28 A. B. C.
16.29 A. B. C. D.
16.30 B.
16.31 G.
16.32 A.
16.33 D.
16.34 H.
16.35 F.
16.36 C.
16.37 I.
16.38 E.

Chapter 17
Quick Quiz:
17.1 B.
17.2 A.
17.3 D.
17.4 C.
17.5 A.
17.6 C.
17.7 B.
17.8 D.
17.9 B.
17.10 C.
17.11 D.
17.12 A.
17.13 D.
17.14 C.
17.15 B.
17.16 A.

Chapter 17
Chapter Quiz
17.1   I.
17.2   A.
17.3   G.
17.4   F.
17.5   B.
17.6   E.
17.7   D.
17.8   C.
17.9   H.
17.10   K.
17.11   C.
17.12   A.
17.13   G.
17.14   H.
17.15   J.
17.16   I.
17.17   E.
17.18   D.
17.19   F.
17.20   B.
17.21   Q37.0
17.22   Q26.3
17.23   Q72.41
17.24   Q55.1
17.25   Q33.3
17.26   Q89.4
17.27   Q62.62
17.28   Q06.1
17.29   Q44.2
17.30   Q16.3
17.31   Q92.0
17.32   C.
17.33   B. C.
17.34   A. B. C. D.
17.35   A. B. C. F.
17.36   A. B. C.
17.37   A. B. C. D.
17.38   B. C. E.

17.39   B. C.
17.40   A. C.

Chapter 18
Quick Quiz
18.1   D.
18.2   C.
18.3   B.
18.4   A.
18.5   D.
18.6   C.
18.7   B.
18.8   A.
18.9   C.
18.10   D.
18.11   B.
18.12   A.
18.13   C.
18.14   A.
18.15   D.
18.16   B.

Chapter 18
Chapter Quiz
18.1   D.
18.2   E.
18.3   A.
18.4   B.
18.5   F.
18.6   C.
18.7   3
18.8   1
18.9   4
18.10   0
18.11   2
18.12   S
18.13   F
18.14   S
18.15   S
18.16   F

18.17   E.
18.18   H.
18.19   O.
18.20   S.
18.21   I.
18.22   M.
18.23   Q.
18.24   F.
18.25   P.
18.26   A.
18.27   D.
18.28   R.
18.29   J.
18.30   K.
18.31   C.
18.32   N.
18.33   L.
18.34   B.
18.35   G.

Chapter 19
Quick Quiz:
19.1   B.
19.2   A.
19.3   D.
19.4   C.

Chapter 19
Chapter Quiz
19.1   S00.01XS
19.2   S36.115D
19.3   S30.1XXA
19.4   S61.052D
19.5   S09.22XA
19.6   S72.471G
19.7   S52.134S
19.8   S01.24XA
19.9   S41.012S
19.10   S02.671A
19.11   A. B. C. D. F. G.

19.12 A. B. C. D. G.	20.9 D.	21.11 A.
19.13 B. C. D. F. G.	20.10 F.	21.12 D.
19.14 A. B. C. D. F. G.	20.11 G.	21.13 B.
19.15 A. B. C. D. F. G.	20.12 A.	21.14 D.
19.16 A. B. C. D. E. G.	20.13 B. E. G.	21.15 C.
19.17 B. C. D. F. G.	20.14 B. C. D. G.	21.16 A.
19.18 A. B. C. D. F. G.	20.15 A. B. C. D. G.	
19.19 B. C. D. G.	20.16 B. C. G.	**Chapter 21**
19.20 A. B. C. D. G.	20.17 A. B. C. D. G.	**Chapter Quiz**
19.21 T28.1XXA	20.18 A. B. C. D. G.	21.1 D.
19.22 T78.01XD	20.19 A. B. G.	21.2 H.
19.23 T67.4XXA	20.20 W54.0XXD	21.3 I.
19.24 T71.121S	20.21 W07.XXXA	21.4 E.
19.25 T20.27XA	20.22 W21.05XA	21.5 M.
19.26 T17.400D	20.23 V23.5XXA	21.6 N.
19.27 T83.032A	20.24 W89.1XXD	21.7 B.
19.28 T15.01XD	20.25 X95.01XS	21.8 F.
19.29 T20.112S	20.26 X15.1XXA	21.9 J.
19.30 T33.811A	20.27 V00.112D	21.10 L.
19.31 T23.672S	20.28 Y63.2	21.11 A.
19.32 T73.1XXA	20.29 X50.1XXD	21.12 M.
19.33 A. B. C. D. E. F.	20.30 X04.XXXA	21.13 G.
19.34 A. B. C. D.	20.31 Y28.1XXS	21.14 C.
19.35 B. C. D. F.	20.32 Y35.212D	21.15 K.
19.36 A. B. C. D. E. F.	20.33 V43.63XA	21.16 A.
19.37 A. B. C. D. F.	20.34 X30.XXXS	21.17 B. C. D.
19.38 Y	20.35 Y92.015	21.18 B. C. D.
19.39 N	20.36 V75.6XXS	21.19 A. B.
19.40 N		21.20 E. F.
19.41 Y	**Chapter 21**	21.21 A. B. C. D.
	Quick Quiz:	21.22 A. B. C.
Chapter 20	21.1 C.	21.23 E.
Chapter Quiz	21.2 A.	21.24 A. B. C. D. E. F.
20.1 I.	21.3 B.	21.25 B. E.
20.2 E.	21.4 D.	21.26 A. C. F.
20.3 C.	21.5 B.	21.27 A. B.
20.4 K.	21.6 C.	21.28 A. B. C.
20.5 H.	21.7 A.	21.29 B. C. D.
20.6 J.	21.8 D.	21.30 B. C. E. F.
20.7 B.	21.9 B.	21.31 B. C.
20.8 L.	21.10 C.	21.32 B.C.

21.33   E.
21.34   C.D.E.F.
21.35   B.C.F
21.36   A.B.D.E.
21.37   C.

Chapter 22
Quick Quiz:
22.1   C.
22.2   A.
22.3   D.
22.4   B.

Chapter 22
Chapter Quiz
22.1   C.
22.2   E.
22.3   A.
22.4   H.
22.5   B.
22.6   I.
22.7   F.
22.8   J.
22.9   D.
22.10   G.
22.11   C.
22.12   E.
22.13   E.
22.14   G.
22.15   A.
22.16   D.
22.17   A.
22.18   H.
22.19   B.
22.20   C.

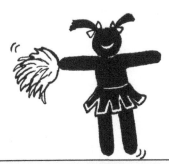

FINAL REVIEW

1. J.	34. D.	67. R79.0
2. R.	35. I.	68. B17.11
3. H.	36. J.	69. O40.2XX0
4. E.	37. S.	70. N11.1
5. M.	38. L.	71. H61.322
6. G.	39. P.	72. A32.0
7. N.	40. M.	73. S90.112D
8. F.	41. M.	74. K35.3
9. S.	42. J.	75. F40.231
10. C.	43. N.	76. T20.13XA
11. K.	44. K.	77. Q25.43
12. A.	45. Q.	78. P72.1
13. D.	46. P.	79. D50.0
14. L.	47. E.	80. G40.319
15. P.	48. R.	81. B.
16. Z.	49. T.	82. A.
17. O.	50. F.	83. C.
18. I.	51. O.	84. E.
19. Q.	52. C.	85. D.
20. H.	53. L.	86. A. B. C. D. E.
21. G.	54. S.	87. B. C. D. F.
22. H.	55. G.	88. A. B. C.
23. A.	56. H.	89. A. B. C. D. F.
24. E.	57. I.	90. A. B. C. D.
25. R.	58. D.	91. B. C. E.
26. Q.	59. A.	92. B. C. D.
27. N.	60. B.	93. B. C. D.
28. O.	61. I20.1	94. A. B. C. D.
29. B.	62. E05.01	95. B. C. D. E.
30. C.	63. L23.3	96. A. B. C. F.
31. K.	64. J20.2	97. A. B. C.
32. F.	65. M60.070	98. A. B. C. D. F.
33. T.	66. H34.8120	

Appendix B

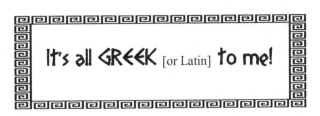

It's all GREEK [or Latin] to me!

On these pages are some of the more common Greek and Latin word parts used in medicine that you'll find in *ICD-10-CM Quick Learn*. The Greek (G) or Latin (L) derivation is followed by the chapter in which the term first appears. This list is a great quick reference when you're stumped by a long, complicated medical term.

a(n) no; not G 3

acute sharp; severe L 9

aden(o) gland G 11

adnexa appendages; accessory parts L 7

affective moods; feelings L 5

-al pertaining to L 14

-algia pain G 8

amnio(n) fetal membrane G 15

angi blood, lymph vessel G 12

angina strangling L 9

ankyl crooked; stiff G 13

ante before; prior to L 15

arterio artery L 9

arthro joint G 13

-ary pertaining to L 9

athero porridge G 9

auricle external ear L 8

bacteria rod G 1

benign good; non-cancerous L 2

bi two L 5

bifida split L 17

blephar eyelid G 7

brady slow G 9

bronch(o) windpipe G 10

bullous bubble L 12

bursa sacs in connecting tissue G 13

carcin cancerous G 2

card(io) heart L 9

calculus pebble L 11

cele tumor; swelling G 14

cephal(o) head; brain G 6

cerebro brain L 6

cerumen ear wax L 8

chole bile G 11

chondr cartilage G 13

choroid skinlike G 7

chronic over time G 9

col(o) colon L 11

con with; together L 7

congenitus born together L 16

conjunctiv join together L 7

cornu horn L 7

cranium skull L 6

cutis skin L 12

cycl circle G 7

cyst sac; bladder G 11

cyto cell G 3

-dactyl finger G 17

derm(a) skin G 12

diverticulum little sac L 11

dorso back L 13

dura hard L 6

-dynia pain G 11

dys bad; difficult G 11

effus(e)(ion) to pour out L 8

embol stopper; plug G 9

-emia blood G 3

encephal(o) head; brain G 6

endo within; inside G 9

enter(o) intestine G 11

epi upon; over G 10

erythema redness G 12

esophag(o) esophagus G 11

extra outside L 6

fissure groove; deep furrow L 11

fistula passage; pipe L 11

gastr(o) stomach G 11

-genesis formation, G 17

-genic arising from; producing G 13

gingivi gums L 11

glomerular little ball L 14

gloss(o) tongue G 11

glottis back of the tongue G 10

glyco sweet G 18

hemi half G 6

hemo(a) blood G 3

hepa(to) liver G 11

hidros sweat G 18

hist tissues; cells G 2

hyper excess; big; enlargement G 3

hypo under; reduced; smaller G 3

-ia disease; condition L 10

-iasis disease; condition G 11

-ic pertaining to G 11

ileus twisting G 11

immun safe L 3

in situ in position localized L 2

infarct dying tissue L 13

interstitium the space between L 10

intra inside L 6

irid(o) iris G 7

ische to hold back G 9

-ism condition G 3

-itis inflammation G 4

kerato horn; cornea G 7

-kinesia movement G 11

labyrinth maze G 8

lacrima tears L 7

laryng(o) larynx G 10

-lex(ia)(is) diction G 18

lith stone G 11

lymph lymphatic system L 2

-lysis breaking down G 13

-lytic breaking down G 3

macro large; big G 17

mal bad L 13

-malacia softening G 7

mamm(a)(o) breast L 14

mast(o) breast G 14

maxilla jawbone L 10

media medium; middle L 8

melan dark G 2

men month G 15

meninges membranes G 6

meniscus crescent shaped G 13

met measure G 7

metra uterus G 14

micro small G 17

mono one G 6

morph form; shape G 2

mye bone marrow G 13

myel spine G 6

myo muscle G 6

myring ear drum L 8

naso nose L 10

natal birth L 16

necr(o) cellular death G 13

neo new G 2

nephr(o) kidney G 14

neur(o) nerve G 6

occlusion close L 13

odont tooth G 11

oligo too small; too few G 14

-ology study of G 2

-oma tumor; swelling G 2

oophor ovaries G 14

-opia sight; vision G 7

opthalm(o) eye G 17

oral mouth L 11

orch testicle G 14

-osis condition G 3

osteo bone G 13

ot ear G 8

pancrea pancreas G 4

papulo pimple L 12

para alongside of G 4

-paresis muscular weakness G 6

partum childbirth L 15

patella small pan L 13

-pathy disease; disorder G 6

pectoris chest L 9

-penia lack G 3

peri around; near G 9

-phagia swallowing G 18

pharyng(o) pharynx G 10

-phasia speech disorder G 18

phle(b) vein G 6

phonia voice G 18

phyte that which grows G 13

pinna feather L 8

-plasia development; formation G 14

-plasm form G 2

-plegia stroke; paralysis G 6

pleur membranes lining lungs G 10

-pnea breath G 16

pneum(o) lungs G 10

polar opposite in character L 5

poly many G 4

por(o) pore G 13

post after; behind L 8

pre prior to L 15

proct(o) anus G 11

psych mind G 5

ptosis drooping G 7

pulmo lungs L 9

pyro fire G 13

quad four L 6

ren(a)(o) kidney L 14

retro behind L 11

rhin(o) nose G 10

rhythmos rhythm G 9

rosaceus rose colored L 12

-rrhage abnormal flow or discharge G 3

-rrhea discharge of pus or fluid G 8

salping(o) tube G 8

scler hard G 7

scoli(o) crooked G 13

sepsis toxins from infection G 15

sequela sequel; following L 9

sial(o) saliva G 11

soma body G 5

sperm(a) seed; sperm G 14

spina thorn; spine L 17

splen spleen G 3

spondyl vertebra G 13

squamous scale-like L 12

sten(o) narrow G 9

stoma mouth G 11

stricture narrowing; constriction L 14

-stomy surgical opening G 11

sub below L 6

suppuratus producing pus L 8

syn together G 17

synov joint fluid L 13

tachy fast G 9

teno tendon G 13

therm heat G 16

thromb(o) clot G 3

trache(o) trachea G 10

tri three L 15

trich(i)(o) hair G 12

troph(y) nourishment G 11

tympano drum (as in ear drum) G 8

ur urine G 14

vascular blood vessels L 6

vesic(o) bladder L 14

virus poison L 1

Visit

quicklearnguides.com

for more information, the latest details and to inquire about quantity discounts.

Also Avalable:

Medical Terminology Quick Learn
The Easiest Guide to
Mastering Basic Medical Terminology
&
Medical Coding Quick Learn
The Easiest Guide to
Mastering Basic Medical Procedure Coding

NOTES...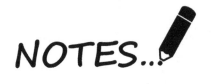

Made in United States
North Haven, CT
18 March 2024

50171560R00235